We Are In This Together

A Woman's Guide to Claiming Her Changes and Power; A Must-Read for Men Wanting to Support and Understand Women

Eda G.

Table of Contents

We Are In This Together 1

Table of Contents 4

Introduction 14

Chapter 1: Navigating Life Through Our Cycles 18

Chapter 2: The Power of Having a Womb 33

Chapter 3: Tuning Into Our Rhythm 50

Chapter 4: Emotional Landscapes 65

Chapter 5: Grandmother Power (Ancient Wisdom) 77

Chapter 6: Our Partners in the Journey 89

Chapter 7: Wellness Practices 106

Chapter 8: Celebrating Every Phase Like a Movement 126

Chapter 9: Creating Supportive Communities 144

Chapter 10: We Are in This Together 162

Conclusion 174

References 180

Table of Contents

Introduction

  Chapter 1: Navigating Life Through Our Cycles

Rhythms of Renewal

  Unveiling the Mysteries: The Four Phases and Their Real-Life Impacts

Syncing With the Symphony

  Tips for Getting Started
  Changes in Each Phase

Embracing the Power Within

  Cultivating Inner Strength
  Personal Stories

Tools for the Journey

  Period-Tracking Apps
  Yoga
  Meditation
  Movement
  Deep Breathing

Call to Action

  Chapter 2: The Power of Having a Womb

The Womb as a Center of Power

  Biological and Physiological Importance of the Womb
  The Womb as the Center for Feminine Energy and Creativity
  The Spiritual Dimension of the Womb
  The Womb as a Source of Feminine Power

The Historical Significance of the Womb

  A Cultural Perspective of the Womb

The Symbolism of the Womb
The Womb in Mythology

Biological Miracles of the Womb

Anatomy of the Womb and Its Physiological Functions
The Role of Hormones
The Role of the Womb in Menstruation
The Role of the Womb in Pregnancy

The Womb and Feminine Identity

The Role of the Womb in the Feminine Identity
The Impact of Emotions on the Womb
How a Healthy Womb Affects Self-Acceptance

Empowering Through Understanding

How Women Perceive and Experience Their Wombs
Self-Care Through Nutrition and Exercise
Warning Signs That Something Is Wrong With the Womb

Harnessing Creative Energy

Creativity and the Womb
Practices to Engage the Creative Potential of the Womb

Celebrating Our Wombs

Rituals and Practices
Yoni Steaming

Conclusion: Embracing Our Inner Strength
Call to Action
Chapter 3: Tuning Into Our Rhythm
Embracing Our Natural Rhythms

Why Rhythm Matters

Understanding Our Body's Cycles

The Science of Rhythms
Menstrual Rhythms

Practical Ways to Sync With Our Rhythms

Daily Habits
Sleep Patterns
Diet and Exercise

Mindfulness and Meditation

Mindfulness Practices
Meditation for Menstrual Health

Integrating Rhythm in Relationships

Communication Strategies
Support Networks

Case Studies and Success Stories

Real-Life Examples
Lessons Learned

To Conclude: Moving Forward in Harmony
Call to Action
Chapter 4: Emotional Landscapes
Embracing Our Inner Seasons
Spring–The Maiden (Post-Menstruation)

New Beginnings and Renewal
Strategies for the Maiden

Summer—The Mother (Ovulatory Phase)

Nurturing Growth and Connection
Living as the Mother

Autumn—The Witch (Pre-Menstruation)

Reflection and Self-Focus
Harnessing the Witch's Power

Winter—The Wise Woman (Menstruation)

Guidance From the Wise Woman

Conclusion: Integrating Our Emotional Cycle
Call to Action
Chapter 5: Grandmother Power (Ancient Wisdom)
Tapping Into Ancestral Wisdom
Wisdom Across Cultures

Common Themes and Lessons

Practical Teachings and Their Applications

Health and Healing
Relationships and Community Building
Spiritual Connections and Rituals—Spiritual Practices Passed Down

Integrating Ancient Rituals Today
Stories of Resilience and Strength—Inspirational Anecdotes

Marisol Kiyoko and Resilience
Chrys Nguyen's Story of Providing Community Care and Support

Conclusion: Embracing the Grandmother Spirit
Moving Forward With Ancient Insights
Chapter 6: Our Partners in the Journey
Building Bridges Together—Understanding Each Other's Rhythms
Communicating Clearly in a Relationship: The Foundation of Understanding
Understanding Together: Navigating the Realities of Our Period and Fostering
Intimacy Through Shared Knowledge
Supporting Each Other

Emotional Support Techniques

Overcoming Challenges Together
Empowering Our Partners

Role of Advocacy
Celebrating Togetherness
Conclusion: Stronger Together
Chapter 7: Wellness Practices
Aligning Everyday Wellness With Our Cycle
Wellness Practices for Each Phase

Spring—Maiden or Virgin Phase Wellness
Summer—Mother Phase Wellness
Autumn—Witch Phase Wellness
Winter—Wise Woman Phase Wellness
Personalized Wellness Practices for Each Phase

Conclusion: Integrating Practices Into Daily Life
Chapter 8: Celebrating Every Phase Like a Movement
Embracing Our Inner Dance
Spring—Celebrating New Beginnings

The Maiden's Awakening
Activities and Celebrations
Rituals Honoring the Maiden

Summer—Embracing Full Bloom

The Mother's Embrace
Activities and Celebrations
Rituals Honoring the Mother

Autumn—Reflecting in the Harvest

The Witch's Wisdom
Activities and Celebrations
Rituals Honoring the Enchantress

Winter—Honoring the Retreat

The Wise Woman's Rest
Activities and Celebrations
Rituals Honoring the Wise Woman

Cultivating a Celebration Mindset

Daily Practices to Honor Each Phase
Mindfulness and Appreciation

Conclusion: A Continuous Cycle of Celebration
Chapter 9: Creating Supportive Communities
The Power of Connection

Building Women Circles

The Foundation of Community: Women Circles and Gatherings

Women Circles: The Bedrock of Our Support Network
Strengthening Bonds
Building Your Extended Community
Nurturing Engagement Within and Beyond—Inviting Members to Our Circle

Fostering Open Communication

Create a Judgment-Free Haven
Organizing Community Activities—Hosting Heart-Centered Women's Gatherings
Leveraging Technology—Digital Tools for Connectivity
Overcoming Challenges—Resolve Conflicts With Compassion
Evaluating Effectiveness

Conclusion: A Continuous Journey
Chapter 10: We Are in This Together
The Universal Nature of Menstrual Experience
Understanding the Impact on All

Direct Impact
Indirect Impact

Building Empathy and Understanding

Education for Everyone
Sharing Stories

Practical Support Systems

In Homes and Families
In Workplaces

Celebrating Togetherness

Cultural Festivals From Around the World That Honor Menstruation
Creating New Traditions to Recognize and Support Menstruation

Conclusion: A Call to Collective Action
Conclusion
Celebrating Our Collective Journey
Recognizing Our Shared Strength
Empowering Ourselves and Others
Envisioning a Supportive Future
Gratitude and a Rallying Cry
References

For Magdalene.

I bow my head in gratitude to this experience called life, which has co-created this book with me as a first step toward freedom for all women. What a surprise this has been. I am deeply grateful to all my teachers and guides, and to the luminaries among us. Thank you to the unknown players who make this infinite game worth playing, and to all those who support my journey and existence. You inspire my expression every day. Thank you. I see you.

Introduction

Every woman you know and love
Every woman you admire from afar
Every frenemy and foe
Chances are you've bled together.
–Nikki Tajiri

No other experience creates an unspoken bond among women as strongly as our shared experience of menstruation—a bond that weaves us together in sisterhood. Regardless of the color of our skin, the scale of our wealth, or the language we speak, the rhythm of our cycles connects us on a basic level. It's like we're all part of this ancient, universal club, linked by the ebb and flow of our bodies' natural cycles. And in that shared experience, there's a sense of solidarity, a feeling that we're all in this together, supporting and understanding each other.

Back in the day, menstruation was revered as a sacred process and regarded as kind of magical. Ancient peoples believed women's periods were connected to the moon, and that they all happened around the same time as the moon's phases. They even used to keep track of their periods by looking at the moon, suggesting a deep-rooted connection between women's cycles and nature's rhythms.

Before we had electricity, the moon's light helped women's periods stay on track, like a natural clock. And even though different cultures have their own ways of dealing with periods, such as rules about not touching certain things or going to certain places, basic ideas about periods have been pretty similar all over the world.

But for a lot of us, talking about periods used to be a big no-no. It's like we were supposed to hide them and feel embarrassed. Many of us felt disgusted by our own blood; when washing our sheets, changing our tampons, or cleaning up a leak on our outfit, there was so much repulsion and shame around it. It took a while for some of us to realize that periods are totally normal and nothing to be ashamed of. It's like flipping a switch from feeling embarrassed to feeling strong and connected to nature's rhythms.

For me, embracing my period means owning the awesome power of being a woman. It's about discovering who I am and accepting myself just the way I am, period and all. It was through my personal journey of shifting from shame to empowerment that the idea for this book was born. I realized that my own transformation had the potential to empower countless others to embrace their menstrual cycles with ceremony and celebration.

And so, with a sense of purpose and passion, I took up the challenge of creating a guide that not only educates but also empowers, inviting women to join me in reclaiming the narrative around menstruation and embracing the natural power of womanhood.

Within the pages of this book, you are invited to start a journey to understand your body's natural rhythms. It's a journey that will reveal the secrets of ancient wisdom regarding menstruation, make our relationships stronger, and help us feel more confident. As we start this journey together, let's recognize how important it is to understand and accept our menstrual cycle. It's not just a bodily thing; it's like a beautiful dance that happens inside us, a cyclical symphony following the rhythms of nature, that takes place every month.

You'll find more than just information; you'll find a movement—a call to all women and the men who stand by their sides to honor and celebrate the innate power of the menstrual cycle. It is a declaration for womanhood, an anthem for those ready to tune into the symphony of their bodies and reclaim their rightful place in the world.

It is an important reminder to you that you are not alone on this journey. *We are in this together*, bound by the shared experience of womanhood and the powerful transformations that occur within us each month. This book is a tribute to the strength of our collective sisterhood and a reminder that, together, we can empower each other to thrive.

Throughout these pages, we will explore the complex seasons of our menstrual cycle, uncovering the hidden wisdom that lies within each phase. From the uplifting energy of ovulation to the soul-searching reflection of menstruation, we will learn how every aspect of our cycle contributes to our overall well-being and personal growth.

Through a blend of science and ancient wisdom, we'll bridge the gap between modern understanding and timeless traditions, discovering how to mix these things together smoothly to make our lives better. Together, we will learn practical strategies to align our daily routines with the different stages of our menstrual cycle, nurturing ourselves, cultivating deeper intimacy in our relationships, and making plans for the week ahead.

And as we journey together, remember that this is not just a book—it is a guide, a companion, and a celebration of womanhood in all its beauty and complexity. It is a tribute to the power of self-care, self-awareness, and self-love and a reminder that by embracing our truth, we can liberate ourselves.

So let's start this journey together, hand in hand, heart to heart, as we honor the sacred ceremony of the movement in our body and embrace our innate power as women.

Chapter 1:
Navigating Life Through Our Cycles

Calling women the miniature earth is not an exaggeration, as we do carry the whole world inside us. Like the moon and the stars, we are cyclical beings living in a 28-day menstrual cycle in harmony with the moon. Much like the rivers of the world wash over the land, the red stream of blood flows from us, washing the debris of dead cells from our bodies. Like the tides of the ocean, our period rises with the moon.

Isn't it strange that our period, which connects us to the natural world, is the only bodily process that carries the burden of shame and secrecy? Especially as our period is a tool for women's empowerment, manifestation, and creation, which is achieved when we harmonize our cycle with the activities in our life through our lifestyle. Historically, ancient cultures revered menstruation, recognizing its deep connection to the lunar cycle and nature's rhythms. This sacred perception has evolved, but understanding these ancient views can help us reconnect with the natural harmony of our cycles today.

There is one organ—the womb—that believes in us more than we believe in ourselves. Every month for 30–40, sometimes 50, years, it decides to create life. Every month, it finds that life force and the call to create life.

Once we understand the highs and lows of our emotional state, our stamina, and our activity level during different phases of our menstrual cycle, we can discover why we feel the way we do and how to get maximum output from ourselves at different times of the month. This self-knowledge will help us own everything our periods bring into our life, empowering us. Self-discovery starts with understanding the phases of our menstrual cycle.

Rhythms of Renewal

You may be surprised to know that, just like we have four seasons and there are four phases of the moon, our menstrual cycle is divided into four phases. Not just that, but the lunar cycle and menstrual cycle both last 28–29 days. Perhaps that is the reason our monthly visitor is called menstruation, derived from the Greek word *mene* or "moon." In all the ancient cultures around the world, this time was called the "moon time" and was associated with renewal as we shed the dead cells from our body. Just as the moon causes tides in the ocean, it affects our menstrual cycle.

Unveiling the Mysteries: The Four Phases and Their Real-Life Impacts

Follicular Phase—Maiden (Virgin): Independence and New Beginnings (Waxing Moon, 7–10 days)

This phase starts right after your period ends and lasts until ovulation. Hormone levels are low to begin with but slowly rise, thickening the uterus lining and leading to ovulation.

This phase is like springtime, bringing new energy and possibilities. Take a moment to reflect: What new projects or ideas have sparked your interest during this phase? Write them down and consider how you can nurture these budding inspirations. After your period, your energy starts to increase as your body prepares for ovulation. This phase, usually lasting a week, is like the early stages of a young plant's growth, filled with new thoughts and small steps forward. You might feel more lively, friendly, and focused, making it an ideal time for getting things done and being active. As the follicular phase concludes, your body transitions into the ovulatory phase, where the energy and growth cultivated during this time reach their peak.

Ovulatory Phase—Mother: Nurturing, Care, and Growth (Full Moon, 3–4 days)

Lasting a few days, this phase is when you're most fertile, making pregnancy possible. Women might feel more attractive and energetic during this time.

This phase is like summer, when you feel super energetic and friendly, especially around ovulation time. Reflect on your social connections and consider how you can strengthen them. Who can you reach out to for collaboration or support? Plan social activities or networking events to maximize this high-energy phase. Celebrate your vitality by engaging in physical activities that challenge you and make you feel alive. You're more likely to want to hang out with others and maybe even think about having a baby. Usually, on about the 13th day of your cycle, you might feel really happy, good-looking, and interested in being intimate. With lots of estrogen around, you feel confident and outgoing, making it easier to connect with people. As the heightened energy of summer begins to wane, your body prepares to move inward, reflecting the autumnal shift into the luteal phase.

Luteal Phase—Enchantress (Witch/Wild Woman): Reflection and Self-Focus (Waning Moon, 10–14 days)

Starting after ovulation, this is the longest phase, ending with your next period. Hormone levels rise, preparing the uterus for pregnancy. Later, hormone levels drop, causing the lining to shed.

This phase is like autumn, a time to look inward and think deeply. Reflect on the progress of your current projects and identify what needs to be completed or refined. This is a great time for detail-oriented tasks and tying up loose ends. Journal about any emotional insights or revelations you experience during this introspective period. Create a cozy, supportive environment for yourself to foster self-reflection and self-care. This is when you might have important conversations with yourself and make decisions. Emotionally, you might feel like finishing things off (tasks, projects, etc.) and paying extra attention to details, as if you're using a magnifying glass. As hormone levels drop, you might feel more quiet, and it's important to take care of yourself and stay calm during this time. With the quiet introspection of autumn giving way to the deep rest of winter, your body naturally flows into the menstrual phase.

Menstrual Phase—Wise Woman (Crone): Insight and Guidance During Menstruation (New Moon, 3–7 days)

This is your period phase, lasting a few days. Hormone levels are low, energy is down, and your body needs rest and nourishment.

This phase feels like winter, giving you a chance to relax and let go. Reflect on the past cycle: What worked well, and what could be improved? Use this time to release any emotional or physical tension. Create a ritual for letting go, such as writing down worries and burning the paper, or practicing deep breathing exercises. Embrace restful activities like reading, gentle yoga, or meditation to recharge your body and mind. Listen to your inner voice and honor the need for solitude and introspection. It's a time to take it easy and think about things, letting your mind wander. Emotionally, your hormones help you understand things without even trying, making this a great time to think deeply and rest a lot. Trusting your feelings and giving yourself time alone is really important during this phase.

Menstruating in sync with the lunar cycle is believed to bring out different qualities. For instance:

- **White moon cycle:** Starting menses with the new moon. Some believe this makes a person more fertile and reflective, and that it is a good time to start new things.

- **Red moon cycle:** Menstruating during the full moon. This is seen as a time to embrace passion, outgoingness, and sexuality—and it's a good time to let go of things.

- **Pink moon cycle:** Beginning menses during the waxing moon. This a time of transition.

- **Purple moon cycle:** Starting menses during the waning moon. This is associated with healing (Walter, 2021).

Syncing With the Symphony

I used to dread my period every month, feeling it was a curse. But once I started tracking my cycle and understanding the changes, I began to see it as a powerful part of who I am. –Unknown

Imagine your body as an orchestra, with each part playing its own instrument. Your menstrual cycle is like the music it creates. Now, think of your lifestyle as the conductor of this orchestra. Just as a conductor guides musicians to play in harmony, your lifestyle choices can help harmonize your menstrual cycle with nature.

We all notice that our feelings and energy change depending on where we are in our cycle. Before our period, we might feel grumpy and tired, but in the middle of our cycle, we might feel full of energy. What if we could adjust what we do, what we eat, and how we think based on where we are in our cycle? That's where "cycle syncing" comes in.

Cycle syncing means adjusting our daily routines to match the natural ups and downs of our hormones during the four phases of our menstrual cycle. For instance, during the follicular phase, we might find that engaging in high-energy activities like cardio workouts is more beneficial, while in the luteal phase, focusing on calming exercises such as yoga or stretching can help maintain balance and reduce stress. This approach is based on the understanding that our needs change depending on where we are in our cycle. Different hormones, like estrogen and progesterone, affect our mood, energy, and how our body works.

To cycle sync, we need to know where we are in our cycle and how our cycle works. Different hormones take charge during each phase, affecting our energy levels and how we feel. This method works best for people who have regular periods. If you're going through menopause or have irregular periods, it might not work well for you; and, of course, it won't apply when you're pregnant.

Cycle syncing helps us connect with how our cycle affects our feelings, energy, and mood. Instead of fighting against our body's natural ups and downs, we work with them. By matching what we do with our energy levels, we can be more productive and avoid feeling burnt out.

Understanding how hormones affect our mood can also help us find ways to feel better and reduce PMS symptoms. Adjusting our exercise routines based on our cycle can also improve how we perform and recover from workouts.

Tips for Getting Started

Cycle syncing starts with tracking our menstrual cycle and how we feel during each phase. We have to make small changes to our lifestyle based on what we learn and listen to our body's signals along the way.

Think of cycle syncing as three main steps:

- **Adapting our activities:** We adjust our daily plans and social events to match our energy and mood.

- **Modifying exercise:** It helps to try different exercises based on where we are in our cycle.

- **Dietary changes:** Eating foods that support our hormonal balance and health throughout our cycle is advised.

Changes in Each Phase

Follicular Phase: Springtime

- **Lifestyle:** The follicular phase is like a fresh start. Stay receptive to fresh concepts, individuals, and experiences.

- **Work and productivity:** This is our creative time! Start fresh projects and allow your creativity to soar.

- **Exercise:** After our period, we feel renewed energy. Try new workouts or activities that excite you.

- **Social life:** Plan fun outings with friends and explore new places together!

Ovulatory Phase: Summer

- **Lifestyle:** You will feel confident and outgoing during this phase.

- **Work and productivity:** Focus on communication and teamwork. This is a great time for presentations and collaborations. Who can you reach out to for collaboration or support? How can you celebrate your vitality and engage in high-energy activities?

- **Exercise:** Your energy is high, so go for more intense workouts if you feel like it.

- **Social life:** Spend extra time socializing and enjoying events with friends.

Luteal Phase: Autumn

- **Lifestyle:** This is the time to finish up tasks and get organized.

- **Work and productivity:** Focus on getting things done and tying up loose ends. What tasks need to be completed or refined?

- **Exercise:** Take it easy with gentler workouts like yoga or strength training.

- **Social life:** You might feel more introverted, so it's okay to take time for yourself. How can you create a supportive environment for self-reflection?

Menstrual Phase: Winter

- **Lifestyle:** Trust your intuition and take care of yourself with rest and self-care activities. What can you release from the past cycle? How can you embrace restful activities and honor the need for introspection?

- **Work and productivity:** Use this time to reflect on your life and what you need.

- **Exercise:** Stick to gentle movements like walking or stretching.

- **Social life:** Enjoy some quiet time alone and listen to your inner voice (Wisner, 2024b).

Embracing the Power Within

Cultivating Inner Strength

Understanding and living in harmony with our menstrual cycle can unlock freedom and self-love for us women. Each woman's cycle is special and gives her valuable feedback about her life. By tuning into our cycle, we can feel empowered and understand our journey each month. Every woman's cycle is unique, and while some feel energized after menstruating, others may feel anxious before their period. However, owning our cycles can help us let go of doubts and realize our true potential.

We can discover the times during our cycle when we can take on extra work and when to step back. Unfortunately, menstruation is often seen as shameful or misunderstood, leading many to hide it or even stop it altogether with products like contraceptive pills. But what if we saw our cycles as a reflection of our health and learned to live in harmony with them? Would it change how we understand ourselves? As a working woman, embracing the power of my menstrual cycle has boosted my self-confidence and made me self-aware.

Personal Stories

Sharing our individual experiences during menstruation is important as we can start a conversation around the subject, encouraging others to stop suffering in silence and letting them be heard. This way, we can empower each other. Here are a couple of women who see their periods as a strength and who are confident enough to share their stories.

Linda, a small business owner, shared her experience in these words: "After trying cycle syncing for a year, my periods are more regular and I experience less intense PMS. This approach has been transformative for me, helping me manage my busy schedule while honoring my body's natural rhythms. I appreciate my body more and feel more connected to myself and my natural rhythm. Cycle syncing helped me understand why my energy, motivation, and emotions change throughout the month. It allows me to flow with these changes and make choices that support my body and health. I don't follow cycle syncing perfectly; instead, I combine it with intuitive and seasonal eating, listening to my body's cravings. Consistency matters more than perfection, making cycle syncing realistic and sustainable. Cycle syncing is a gentle guide, not a strict rulebook. Try different things and discover what suits you best!"

Deborah, a software developer, shares her experience: "Since becoming more aware of my menstrual cycle, I've learned that I'm most productive during my premenstrual phase when my intuition is strong. However, I can feel overwhelmed in the phase right after my period when I'm full of ideas. Taking care of myself and setting boundaries is important during this time. During menstruation, I find that being quiet and still helps me make important connections within myself and with my work projects."

By sharing our experiences, we hope to inspire other women to embrace menstruation as a natural part of life. Let's break the taboo, celebrate our ability to thrive through these changes, and empower everyone to talk openly about periods.

Tools for the Journey

To make the journey of synchronizing our lifestyle and our monthly cycle easier, there are various tools and methods available, including period-tracking apps, meditation techniques, yoga, and breathing exercises.

Period-Tracking Apps

These are changing how women manage their health by providing detailed insights into their menstrual cycles. They predict ovulation, identify patterns, and help women make informed decisions about their bodies:

- **Opening up conversations about women's health:** These apps break taboos around menstruation by encouraging open discussions. They create a supportive community for talking about women's health issues openly and informatively.

- **Enhancing fertility awareness and family planning:** For women trying to conceive or avoid pregnancy, these apps are invaluable. They accurately predict fertile windows and ovulation days, helping women plan their family naturally and effectively.

- **Bridging gaps in women's healthcare services:** In areas with limited healthcare access, period-tracking apps offer a solution.

- **Personalized reminders and resources:** These apps offer reminders for medication, appointments, and self-checks (*How Are Period Tracking Apps,* n.d.).

Top Period-Tracking Apps

To help you choose the right one, here's a quick comparison of the top period-tracking apps, highlighting their unique features and benefits:

- **Clue:** Clue, a free Berlin-based app for women's health, goes beyond menstruation to help users understand their body's cycles. Unique features: Comprehensive health tracking, customizable alerts. Benefits: A deeper understanding of your body's cycles beyond just menstruation.

- **Flo:** Flo's mission is to improve female health using AI to track periods, ovulation, and over 70 symptoms. It can be paired with a partner's device so they can follow our cycles. Unique feature: AI-powered insights, symptom tracking. Benefits: Plan your family naturally and effectively.

- **Luna:** Luna supports teen health by educating and empowering them to understand their cycles and seek support when needed. Unique features: Teen health education, user-friendly interface. Benefits: Empower teens with cycle knowledge.

- **Femble:** Femble is an AI-powered health assistant offering personalized guidance and support for women's health needs. Unique features: Personalized health assistant, expert guidance. Benefits: Tailored support for women's health needs.

- **WomanLog:** This is an easy-to-use period-tracking app with features for tracking pregnancy and menopause. Unique features: Pregnancy and menopause tracking. Benefits: Easy-to-use tracker for all life stages (*The 5 Best Period Tracking Apps,* 2024).

Yoga

Yoga supports women through the different phases of our menstrual cycle and can be adapted to our energy levels, which naturally vary each day. Aligning our yoga practice with our energy levels helps prevent overexertion and depletion. Practicing yoga also helps ease menstrual discomfort and distress by using specific poses that relieve cramps and reduce the severity and duration of discomfort.

As a long-time Kundalini yoga teacher and Yin yoga practitioner, I highly recommend that all women practice dropping deep into their bodies and explore the limits, boundaries, and sensations within themselves regularly.

Meditation

Too much stress affects our hormones, especially during our period. Stress triggers cortisol, which can disrupt our reproductive hormones, causing irregular cycles. Meditation helps lower cortisol levels, reducing stress. Mindfulness meditation involves long, deep breathing, especially with one hand on our womb and the other on our heart, sitting up or lying down. It also helps manage premenstrual stress and emotions. Plus, regular meditation boosts self-esteem and overall well-being.

As it's not easy in today's world, where there's so much external distraction, to silence the mind and go deep in ourselves, I suggest Kundalini yoga's active meditations and chanting as another powerful way to bring awareness to our state of being.

Movement

Pilates combines strength and flexibility to boost our core strength and pelvic stability, harmonizing with the gentle, reflective energy of our menstrual cycles. Just as the moon waxes and wanes, our bodies benefit from exercises that respect and align with these natural rhythms. This can ease period pain and make our cycles more regular. Moves like the pelvic curl and leg slide are great. Additionally, incorporating Kegel exercises, nonlinear movement such as ecstatic dance, and other practices like ectatic dance can further enhance this experience. Kegel exercises can be done daily, with apps available for guidance. Nonlinear movements, especially those that focus on hip opening, are excellent for aligning our mind and body during this time. Ectatic dance is another powerful way to connect with our bodies and promote overall well-being.

Deep Breathing

Diaphragmatic breathing and muscle relaxation can lower stress. Stress affects hormones, so managing it helps regulate our cycles. Long, deep breathing is one of the simplest and most powerful ways to manage anxiety and confusion.

Call to Action

Let's begin our journey of empowerment by embracing our truth and practicing how we can share our experience, making our period a topic of conversation:

- Start a journal or use an app to help you understand your body better. Note your energy level, cravings, and activities to see patterns over time. Here's a simple action plan to get you started:

1. Track your cycle: Choose a period-tracking app and start logging your menstrual cycle and symptoms.
2. Reflect daily: Spend five minutes each day journaling about your mood, energy levels, and any physical sensations.
3. Join a support group: Find or start a local or online group where you can share experiences and gain support.
4. Set monthly goals: At the start of each cycle, set small, achievable goals that align with your energy and mood during each phase.

- Include your partner and join support groups for more understanding.

• Take steps toward self-awareness and empowerment.

Together, let's celebrate our bodies and create a more supportive and informed community.

Chapter 2:
The Power of Having a Womb

The Womb as a Center of Power

As women, our wombs are like gateways to the magic of the universe. They're our direct link to spirituality. It's incredible that life comes from us—it's like a miracle. Reflect on this: How does this miraculous capability make you feel about your own body? Every month during our periods, we let go of things we don't need anymore and get a fresh start. Our wombs are where ideas, dreams, art, humans, and passions grow. Think about a recent project or idea you've nurtured. How did it grow within you before coming to life? Everything in this world is created in a womb, and we're so lucky to have one.

Biological and Physiological Importance of the Womb

The womb is an important organ in our body, shaped like a light bulb or an upside-down pear and about the size of our fist. It has two horn-like parts at the top called fallopian tubes, and it connects to the cervix—the part that expands during delivery—at the bottom. Here are its main jobs:

- **Pregnancy:** The womb grows to accommodate a baby during pregnancy and helps push the baby out during birth.

- **Fertility:** The womb is where a fertilized egg attaches and grows into a baby.

- **Menstrual cycle:** The womb sheds its lining during menstruation, causing bleeding. This cyclical process, referred to as the "creatrix," symbolizes the womb's creative and life-giving power, connecting us to the cycle of life and our role in creation. It serves as a reminder of our interconnectedness with the natural world and our connection to Mother Earth.

Our womb also supports our bladder, bowel, and pelvic organs. It has networks of blood vessels and nerves that supply blood to the pelvis and genitals, including the ovaries, vagina, labia, and clitoris, which are important for sexual pleasure. The womb is essential for experiencing uterine orgasm, and these orgasms activate the cervix (Mandal, 2023). It is also believed that the cervix is the gateway to other dimensions, as we produce DMT when we have these orgasms. DMT, or N-dimethyltryptamine, is produced in women in the cervix, especially during natural birth or cervical orgasms. This can lead to phenomena like orgasmic birth, where DMT activation during orgasm induces otherworldly feelings and potentially transcendental states. The cervix is a portal for healing, pleasure, and orgasm, revealing its potential significance.

The Womb as the Center for Feminine Energy and Creativity

Our womb is more than just a body part; it's the sacred center of our feminine essence and holds deep meaning. *Womb energy* refers to everything about our womb and reproductive system, physically, emotionally, and spiritually. Physically, it affects our health, vitality, and fertility, including our ovaries, while the emotional and spiritual aspects are tightly connected to our womb's health. Spiritually, womb energy is about the power within us, affecting how we connect in relationships, stay grounded, set boundaries, experience pleasure, and express creativity—not just in making babies but also in art and ideas. Our womb is key to our energy, and tapping into it can lead to healthier relationships and more fulfilling lives.

The Spiritual Dimension of the Womb

The womb is a center of deep awareness and wisdom. When we connect with our womb, we tap into our intuition and spiritual connection, even communicating with our future child's soul. During pregnancy, we absorb emotional memories from our mothers and ancestors. It's important to clear these emotions in preparation for bringing new life into the world. *Womb awakening* helps free the traumas and emotional pain of our ancestors so our children can start afresh, without carrying this burden.

The Womb as a Source of Feminine Power

Our womb is closely connected to our emotions, familial lineage, and past experiences. It's where life begins and the maternal bond takes root, symbolizing the nurturing essence of the universe. Associated with feminine energy, it mirrors nature's cycles and offers intuitive wisdom. Embracing its power brings a deeper connection to femininity and purpose. Neglecting emotional aspects can lead to physical issues like pain during intercourse, emphasizing the importance of holistic creativity. Trauma can disrupt the womb's energy, resulting in fertility issues. *Womb healing* restores balance, promoting emotional well-being and self-love.

The Historical Significance of the Womb

A Cultural Perspective of the Womb

The womb holds great significance across cultures, and this is often reflected in its names, such as *cihuatl* for woman and *nantli* for mother in Nahuatl. It's viewed symbolically as a container, a vase, or even a prison, referring to creativity and womanhood. These varied interpretations show how differently various cultures perceive it, from seeing it as a place of creation to one of decay. In some traditions, the womb symbolizes the universe's growth and change, while in others it's linked to enlightenment and bodily control, especially regarding fluids. Men also attribute creative power to the womb, as shown in religious texts referring to God's womb and using childbirth to explain spiritual concepts like baptism and the church as a mother.

The Symbolism of the Womb

The womb, often symbolized as a cave, represents the Great Mother and embodies fertility and abundance. Throughout history, women have been depicted in complex ways, from nurturing figures to monstrous beings, reflecting societal fears of female sexuality and power. These portrayals influenced perceptions of women as obedient and pure, reinforced through fairy tale tropes like the helpless maiden waiting for a prince to rescue her (Onega, 2021).

The Womb in Mythology

The womb has featured in the mythologies of almost all ancient cultures. For example, in the Sumerian tale "Enki and Ninmah," lesser gods complained to the primeval mother Namma about their hard work creating the earth. Namma asked her son Enki, the god of wisdom, to help. She then made humans by shaping clay in her womb.

Isis, a protector in Egyptian mythology, is often shown with large wings and was seen as Egypt's throne. She took on the qualities of many goddesses, including being a mother figure and ruler of the underworld.

Metaformic theory, proposed by Judy Grahn, suggests that menstruation played a big role in early human culture and rituals. Claude Lévi-Strauss thought that myths from North and South America showed men's fears of chaos if women's periods weren't synchronized.

In ancient Rome, it was believed that a menstruating woman could stop hailstorms and lightning. Mayan mythology says menstruation started as punishment for breaking marriage rules.

In early modern Europe, people thought a woman's womb needed to be just right for fertility and that warmth was important for conception (Onega, 2021).

Biological Miracles of the Womb

Anatomy of the Womb and Its Physiological Functions

The womb is about 2.4–3.1 inches (6–8 centimeters) long and 0.8–1.1 inches (2 to 3 centimeters) wide, and is broader at the top than at the bottom. It has four main parts:

- **the fundus** at the top, where the fallopian tubes connect
- **the body**, which is the main part
- **the isthmus**, which is the narrow part at the bottom
- **the cervix**, which is linked to the vagina

The opening of the womb connects to the vaginal space, forming what is often referred to as the birth canal. Inside the womb is a lining called the endometrium, whose thickness changes during the menstrual cycle. If an egg is fertilized, it attaches here and starts to grow. If not, the lining sheds during menstruation. The endometrium also makes fluids that help sperm and eggs stay alive.

The womb wall is made up of three layers of muscle tissue, with blood vessels and other fibers woven in. This muscle expands during pregnancy and returns to normal after birth, though slightly larger than before (Mandal, 2023).

The Role of Hormones

There are four hormones involved in our reproductive functions, two of which affect the ovaries and indirectly influence the womb:

- **follicle-stimulating hormone (FSH)**, which helps eggs mature in the ovaries

- **luteinizing hormone (LH)**, which triggers egg release

The other two hormones directly affect the womb:

- **estrogen** and **progesterone**, which help maintain the lining of the uterus

These hormones, produced by the ovaries, are important for sexual development and for preparing the uterine lining to support fertilized eggs during pregnancy. Estrogen helps with ovulation, growth of the uterine lining, and development of female characteristics like breast growth and wider hips. Progesterone also helps with uterine lining growth and prevents further release of eggs during pregnancy. Any changes in estrogen and progesterone levels can affect our reproductive health and overall well-being (Mandal, 2023).

The Role of the Womb in Menstruation

In a normal period, the lining of the womb gets ready for a potential pregnancy. Small blood vessels grow in the lining, making it thicker and full of blood. If an egg isn't implanted after fertilization, the womb gets rid of this lining through menstruation.

The Role of the Womb in Pregnancy

The womb has three main jobs during pregnancy:

- **Implantation:** Here, a fertilized egg attaches to the lining of the womb, where the placenta starts to grow.

- **Gestation:** The womb gets bigger and thinner as the baby grows inside it, making room for the baby and the fluid around it.

- **Labor:** The womb starts practicing contractions, getting ready for childbirth. These contractions start off mild, like period cramps, but become stronger during labor to push the baby out. After birth, the uterus keeps contracting to push out the placenta and shrink back to its normal size, stopping any bleeding (Mandal, 2023).

The Womb and Feminine Identity

The Role of the Womb in the Feminine Identity

The idea of what it means to be a woman is shaped by social roles like motherhood, family relationships, and domestic duties; these are all related to nurturing, which comes from the womb.

One aspect that is linked to a woman's sense of satisfaction with herself is how well her womb functions. The womb is seen as a symbol of femininity and fertility, and is surrounded by cultural myths and beliefs. The womb also plays a role in how healthy we feel ourselves to be, as it reminds us of its presence through our menstrual cycle.

If we need to have our womb removed, we might feel like we are losing a vital part of ourselves—one that's seen as essential to our identity as a woman.

The Impact of Emotions on the Womb

Our emotions deeply affect our womb. Feelings like shame, fear, and disconnection, especially from traumatic events, can get stuck in our womb, causing blockages. When we push these emotions down, they don't go away; instead, they stay in our womb, causing physical symptoms and emotional pain and making us feel disconnected from our feminine side.

When we experience trauma, our body reacts by tensing up, which can lead to physical and emotional pain, especially in our womb and pelvic area. The trauma's energy gets trapped in our pelvis, causing various symptoms like pain, tension, anxiety, depression, and struggles with intimacy.

How a Healthy Womb Affects Self-Acceptance

Womb healing can bring significant changes to our body, mind, and spirit. What emotions do you associate with your womb, and how can you start healing them?

Emotionally, we shed the weight of disconnection and shame, embracing self-love and acceptance, often as a result of womb healing. Our womb's wisdom guides us toward fulfillment and purpose, offering clarity and insight. Take a moment to meditate on what your womb might be trying to tell you about your current life path.

Spiritually, our womb becomes a channel for strong connection, aligning us with the natural world and the divine feminine. We feel supported by the universe's rhythms, experiencing a deep sense of oneness. We rediscover the power and radiance of our feminine soul, emerging as spiritually attuned beings, fully connected to our essence.

Empowering Through Understanding

How Women Perceive and Experience Their Wombs

Listen to the story of our sister Jin Ae, a Korean immigrant. I hope you find it inspiring how she embraced her femininity. How can your own experiences inspire others? Share your story with a friend, or journal about it.

"As I grew up, I wasn't aware of what it meant to be a girl or to act like one. All I knew was that my mom preferred me to wear pinks and sparkly clothes, telling me that pants were for boys and that girls wore skirts. I was told not to be too friendly with boys to retain my purity. When I grew up and moved to Canada, I thought of working as a chef, as I had learned from seeing my mother cook; however, to my surprise, I found it difficult to be accepted for kitchen jobs at most restaurants, as women were considered too weak to handle the pressure of a busy kitchen. I felt heartbroken and angry that women were supposed to cook at home but not in a restaurant. But I refused to give up, and instead of cursing my womanhood, I got connected with my femininity, owned it fully, and found strength in my identity as a woman to knock at a few more doors—and eventually succeeded."

Self-Care Through Nutrition and Exercise

Exercise

Regular exercise is key for women's reproductive health. What small changes can you start with today? Consider adding yoga or stretching to your daily routine. These activities help maintain hormonal balance, regulate our menstrual cycles, reduce stress, and improve fertility. Aim for 15–45 minutes of exercise a day, like dancing, Kundalini or Yin yoga, stretching, Pilates, gyrotonic training, gyrokinesis, swimming, or walking, followed by 8–11 minutes of meditation, at least 3–4 times a week.

Exercise reduces stress hormones and boosts happy hormones. It also enhances blood flow to the womb, improves insulin levels, and helps manage flexibility and weight, all of which are important for fertility. Additionally, exercise has a positive influence on hormones such as endorphins, serotonin, and dopamine, further contributing to overall well-being and reproductive health. Finally, exercise lifts mood and reduces depression and anxiety, which can affect menstrual cycles and fertility.

Diet and Nutrition

A healthy womb is not just about menstrual cycles and fertility; it's about nurturing our body to maintain hormonal balance, supporting ovulation, and ensuring overall wellness. A balanced diet rich in nutrients like folate, iron, and omega-3 fatty acids is necessary for a healthy womb. Try incorporating one new nutrient-rich food into your meals this week and see it makes you feel.

Foods like leafy greens, berries, eggs, Greek yogurt, nuts, seeds, and beans are good for the womb and overall wellness. Moreover, incorporating herbal supplements such as fenugreek, shatavari, and tongkat ali can be beneficial for reproductive health and hormonal balance. Including lean protein sources in our diet helps regulate our menstrual cycle and promotes healthy egg production for fertility.

Warning Signs That Something Is Wrong With the Womb

If your periods change a lot, see a holistic gynecologist. Make a list of the symptoms or changes you've noticed, as this can help your doctor provide better care. Heavy bleeding or missing periods could mean health issues like hormone imbalances or PCOS. Pelvic pain that won't go away, especially during periods or sex, should also be checked by a doctor. Strange vaginal discharge or new sexual discomfort needs attention, too. If you feel itching or burning around your vagina, it's best to see a gynecologist. These symptoms might be infections that need treatment (Boga, n.d.).

Harnessing Creative Energy

Creativity and the Womb

The womb serves as a creative hub because it's where new life is formed and cared for; it's where natural creative energy brings forth the development of a new person. Womb healing for creatives focuses on reconnecting with the creative energy and intuition within the womb, and involves releasing emotional or energetic blocks that obstruct creativity through practices like meditation, energy healing, journaling, and visualization. Addressing past traumas is essential for fully embracing creativity. The womb, where new life is nurtured, symbolizes the feminine's creative power, extending beyond physical creation to emotional and spiritual realms.

Practices to Engage the Creative Potential of the Womb

To release the creative potential of the womb, a mix of hypnosis and shamanic healing is practiced. These practices help release emotional blocks stored in the womb, which can improve both physical and emotional health by dealing with past traumas and breaking old patterns. Each session is personalized and might include meditation and energy work.

The womb is incredibly powerful, not just for creating babies but also for creativity, healing, and relationships. Unfortunately, this power is often ignored or underestimated. Through meditation, we can tap into the special energy stored in the womb, making it a sacred place of healing and creativity. Meditation teaches us to channel the energy from our womb to our hearts, raising it to a divine level and cleansing our bloodstream. This quickly leads to enlightenment. Once women have learned this redirection, they can practice it whenever they choose. To fully embrace these practices, it's best to be in nature and avoid modern distractions. Even small groups meeting monthly in a natural setting can begin this transformation (Beyk, 2021).

Celebrating Our Wombs

Rituals and Practices

Our first period, or menarche, shapes our view of feminine power, body wisdom, and sacredness. How we are welcomed into womanhood influences our connection with other women, ourselves, and our lineage. Many girls don't receive the honor and wisdom they deserve during their first periods. *Womb rites* aim to reimagine menarche through sharing, learning, creativity, and ceremony within sisterhood.

Ancient cultures revered the womb as a woman's power center. Menstruation was seen as a magical time when a woman's senses were heightened, allowing them to offer wisdom to the community. Some societies have menstrual rituals as empowering spaces. For instance, among the Kalash people in Pakistan, the menstrual house is revered as sacred and serves as a center for women's solidarity. Various religious and cultural ceremonies also honor women during pregnancy, such as *Simantonnayana* in Hinduism and Blessingway ceremonies in modern paganism (Couto-Ferreira & Verderame, 2018).

Yoni Steaming

Yoni steaming is a ritual that honors the womb and its physical source. Originating from ancient China and Mayan culture, it involves sitting over an herbal steam bath to cleanse and support the external vaginal areas. This practice nurtures the sacred site, soothing both physical and emotional trauma. Yoni, a Sanskrit term, refers to the female reproductive organs and is often associated with the divine feminine energy. Women steam to unlock the magic of the womb and the divine feminine within, promoting the well-being of their sexual organs as well as the anus. Yoni steaming in a squatting position aids in bringing the cervix down, allowing the steam to reach it. Additionally, the prolonged sitting period (minimum 15 minutes) allows the steam to benefit the anus as well, which is particularly helpful in cases of hemorrhoids.

Directions for Steaming

Pour water and herbs into a pot. Here, I suggest first mixing the herbs with a pinch of salt, preferably in a wooden bowl. While mixing, put your prayers and intentions into these herbs, asking for what you desire. Then, boil the water in a kettle and pour it over the herbs. Allow them to sit for a minute or two before covering and simmering for 10–15 minutes. The suggested herbs include fresh rosemary, dried lavender, chamomile, calendula, vervain, blue lotus, and roses, with roses being particularly significant due to their high vibrational energy as female flowers.

1. Remove from the heat and allow to cool for five minutes.
2. Test the steam with your hand—it should feel like a comfortable sauna.
3. Place the potholder under the yoni chair and put the pot of steamy herbs on top. Alternatively, place the pot on the floor and do a child's pose or tabletop pose over it, with pillows for support. Chairs are only recommended for those with knee or related issues. Here's what I suggest: You can cover the bowl with a towel to prevent burns from accidental contact. When you assume a comfortable child's pose, you can also cover the lower part of your body with a towel to contain the steam. This posture allows you to sink into your hips, facilitating the opening of your inner thighs to the lower back, enabling the steam to penetrate more deeply and providing a richer experience.
4. Wrap the towel or blanket around your waist, and sit over the hole with your lower back over the pot.

5. Breathe deeply and imagine the herbs cleansing and soothing your body, mind, and spirit.
6. Steam for 15–30 minutes without distractions, if possible accompanied by mantras and prayers.
7. After steaming, move slowly, drink water or herbal tea, and enjoy the therapeutic benefits. Also, you can take a bit of organic castor oil in your hand and wipe it over your yoni. Then, do not wash; it's preferable to do this at night before sleeping. It's also preferable to keep the steam bowl in your bedroom overnight, allowing the flowers to continue working their magic while you sleep. In the morning, you can give the water from the bowl to your plants (*The Ritual & Benefits of Yoni Steaming,* 2023).

Conclusion: Embracing Our Inner Strength

Having a womb is a big part of being a woman. It's where life is created, but it's more than that. In ancient times, people saw the womb as a sacred place for spiritual connection, intuition, and vitality. By connecting with our womb, we can tap into our inner power and heal ourselves and others. Think about a time when you felt truly connected to your body. What made that moment special?

The womb's creative energy helps us make decisions, start new things, and build relationships. What creative project are you working on right now that benefits from this energy? The womb affects our emotional, mental, and spiritual health, guiding us to listen to our bodies and find balance. Taking care of our womb energetically and physically can strengthen our emotional well-being.

When we focus on clearing and cleansing our womb with intention, it can significantly boost our energy and sexual pleasure. A clean and strong womb chakra empowers us to improve our relationships and fulfill our desires. Regularly filling ourselves with our own sensual energy and life force helps us achieve our goals more easily, as our creative center is free from obstacles.

Call to Action

- Join the conversation! Participate in discussions or join groups centered around women's health.

- Start keeping a journal to stay on top of your womb health. Document your feelings, physical changes, and insights. How can this practice enhance your connection with your body? Explore more about your womb health by learning and engaging continuously and manifesting with its creative power.

- Get involved in online forums, local health workshops, or discussion groups to build community engagement and support. Find a local women's health group and attend a meeting. What did you learn from others' experiences? Consider joining a yoni steaming circle or creating one for your community so you can connect with like-minded individuals and share experiences in a supportive environment.

- Let's empower each other to prioritize and take charge of our well-being!

Chapter 3:
Tuning Into Our Rhythm

Embracing Our Natural Rhythms

Nature's rhythms offer stability and harmony, which are evident in the changing seasons, each one bringing unique experiences. Spring brings renewal, while summer offers energy. Autumn signals change, and winter provides stillness. Understanding these cycles helps us live in harmony with nature, leading to a more balanced life. In this chapter, we will explore some tips for embracing these rhythms to improve our well-being.

Why Rhythm Matters

There are so many good reasons to sync up with nature's rhythms. Nature teaches us a lot, and when we pay attention to its patterns, we learn about ourselves and our place in the world. In our fast-paced lives, it's easy to forget to slow down and connect with nature, but doing so can really ground and refresh us. Here's why:

- **Sleep better:** Our bodies naturally follow the day-and-night cycle. By sticking to this rhythm—like avoiding screens before bed and waking up with the sun—we can sleep better and feel more rested. New research advises women to aim for at least eight hours of sleep a night (one hour longer than men) and to even consider an additional hour during our period (Pacheko & Callender, 2024).

- **Feel happier:** Spending time outside and noticing the seasons, plants, colors, and clouds changing can make us feel better. Being in green spaces and observing nature can lower stress and make us happier. And feeling the seasons change helps us feel more connected to the world.

- **Get more done:** When we work with nature's rhythms, we can work smarter. Taking breaks to move around and having an additional glass of water and a change of scenery during the day can keep us from burning out and help us think more creatively.

- **Stay healthy:** Following nature's rhythms can help us develop healthier habits, like eating foods that are clean, locally produced, organic, and in season. If we live in a place where we are not able to get outside, we can use air ionizers, especially those that utilize natural sources such as seaweed. When we live in tune with the seasons and make conscious choices about our environment, our bodies and minds feel their best.

Overall, living in harmony with nature's rhythms is a great way to feel more connected to ourselves and the world around us. So, why not take a moment to step outside and notice what's happening in nature?

Understanding Our Body's Cycles

The Science of Rhythms

Biological rhythms such as our sleep–wake cycle are controlled by our internal clock, called our *circadian rhythm*. This clock manages our body's functions, such as when we sleep and wake up, and even our hormone levels. It's like our body's natural timer. Our brain sends signals throughout the day to keep our body ticking along. Our habits, like when we eat and how much light we're exposed to, can keep these rhythms in check or throw them off-balance. Disrupting these rhythms can mess with our health.

Different rhythms have different cycles—some last a day, others less, and some even a month or a year. Light, exercise, hormones, and medications can all affect these cycles.

Our sleep–wake cycle is the most noticeable rhythm. During the day, our body gets signals to stay awake. As it gets darker, our body starts producing melatonin, which helps us sleep.

But these rhythms aren't just about sleep. They affect things like our metabolism, our heart rate, and our immune system, and they're linked to mental health and diseases. So, keeping our rhythms in sync is pretty important for our overall well-being (*Natural Rhythms,* 2024).

Menstrual Rhythms

Are you wondering how the biological cycles mentioned earlier are related to our menstrual cycle? Well, don't keep guessing! Let's jump right into it:

- **Circadian rhythm and menstrual cycle interaction:** Imagine our body has two clocks: one that tracks our daily rhythms (circadian rhythm) and another that follows our monthly cycle (menstrual rhythm). These two clocks work together and affect each other. Changes to our daily rhythms, like those from working late shifts, can throw our menstrual cycle off-balance.

- **Temperature changes and other rhythms during the menstrual cycle:** After we ovulate (release an egg), our body temperature goes up a bit, but it doesn't rise and fall as much as usual. This temperature change isn't the only thing that shifts during our cycle. Other rhythms in our body, like the ones controlled by hormones such as melatonin and cortisol, might also be affected. Sleep quality usually deteriorates during our period, but our sleep pattern stays pretty consistent throughout our cycle.

● **Impact of disrupted rhythms:** When our daily rhythms get thrown off, it can cause problems with our menstrual cycle, making it irregular. It might also increase our susceptibility to breast health issues. Understanding how these rhythms connect can help us figure out why our moods change during our periods and how it affects our fertility (WebMD Editorial Contributors, n.d.-a).

Practical Ways to Sync With Our Rhythms

The shifts in our body during our period affect appetite, sleep, and mood. Cycle syncing involves adjusting our eating and exercise habits accordingly. Not everyone follows the same formula, but you'll notice patterns over time and get to know what works for you.

Daily Habits

At the start of our cycle, during our winter when we are bleeding, our womb sheds its lining and we might feel tired and need to rest. This is a time for nurturing and slowing down. Create a cozy space for yourself with candles and soft music. Take a warm bath (with Epsom salt, magnesium flakes, or rose petals), read a book that will help you offload, or just chill and be in your own presence. Reflect on what makes you feel most nurtured and incorporate those elements into your self-care routine. Listen to your body—if you're tired, remember that it's okay to take time to rest.

In the next phase, the spring phase, we feel more energetic. It's a good time to set goals, plan for the upcoming weeks, schedule our social interactions, and get creative with activities like painting or writing. We can also keep a moon journal to draw and express our feelings in our spring.

When we reach the summer of our cycle, we feel strong, confident, and resourceful. This is the time to take care of our appearance and try new things, like exploring new places or activities. In our summer, we should connect with others, build relationships, and get involved in groups and gatherings.

As we move into the autumn phase, our energy may decrease and we may feel moody. It is better to practice stress-relief techniques like meditation or aromatherapy during this period. Another option is to take time for ourselves to reflect and create a peaceful environment in our homes.

Sleep Patterns

Changes in hormones during our menstrual cycle can affect how well we sleep. Some of us feel we sleep better when we're ovulating. This better sleep might be because of the higher levels of estrogen.

During the autumn phase, many of us might experience waking up more frequently during the night and having less deep sleep. Typically, sleep quality tends to decline during the middle to late part of this phase. To find comfort during this period, the following activities can be helpful: going to bed early, wearing comfortable and warm clothing, using heavy blankets, drinking calming tea, applying magnesium oil to our feet, listening to binaural beats or sleeping-frequency music, sound baths, and sound healing. Reflect on which practices bring you the most comfort and peace and make them a regular part of your bedtime routine.

Our sleep quality can also mess with our cycle length. If we sleep poorly, don't get enough sleep, or have big changes in our sleep patterns (like when we travel to different time zones), our periods might end up longer or shorter than usual. Plus, sleeping badly is connected to having heavier periods.

Diet and Exercise

Here are some handy tips to sync our eating habits and activity level with the phases of our monthly cycle.

During our period, let's opt for healthy foods like leafy greens and beans to provide comfort and replenish lost nutrients, especially iron. Warm foods such as soups, for example miso soup, can also be beneficial. Additionally, drinking plenty of water can aid our bodies in cleansing themselves. Engaging in gentle exercises like Yin yoga, stretching, or short walks can help alleviate discomfort without overexerting ourselves. Reflect on how these dietary and exercise choices impact your well-being and adjust them to suit your needs.

In the time after our period, we should do light exercises like walking fast, jogging, or dancing to match our body's energy. Eating lots of colorful fruits, veggies, and whole grains will keep up our energy.

When we're ovulating, we should challenge ourselves with intense workouts like cardio or strength training to make the most of our strength, and eat foods with fiber and vitamin B to help with any stomach issues.

During the luteal phase, calming activities like yoga or gentle stretching are best. We should eat foods with magnesium, like leafy greens and nuts, to feel better emotionally and choose complex carbs to keep our energy steady.

Mindfulness and Meditation

Mindfulness Practices

Mindfulness means living in the present moment, paying attention to our thoughts, feelings, and what's around us. When we're mindful of nature, we notice its rhythms—the changing seasons, the wind's sound, the earth's scent. By tuning into nature, we also tune into ourselves, helping us manage stress and feel better overall.

Connecting with nature's elements, like water or trees, can bring peace. Spending time near a lake or river can calm us, while being around trees can ground us. The following mindfulness techniques are helpful throughout our cycle:

• **Mindful walking:** Walking mindfully is a way to ease anxiety and stress. Pay attention to the sensations in your feet as they make contact with the ground, the movement of your legs, and the rhythm of your breath. If you find your mind wandering, gently bring your focus back to the act of walking. Reflect on how this practice makes you feel and incorporate it into your routine when you need a moment of calm.

• **Visualization:** Visualizing a peaceful scene, like a beach or forest, can also help. Close your eyes, imagine the details, and focus on them. If your mind drifts, gently return to your scene.

• **Mindful breathing:** Breathing mindfully is very effective for stress. Focus on your breath and how it feels coming in and out. If your mind wanders, gently bring it back to your breath.

Meditation for Menstrual Health

Meditation can be more effective in relieving stress if it is tailored to our mood and energy level at any given phase of our menstrual cycle.

Phase 1: Menstrual

During this phase, our body is working hard to shed menstrual blood, making us feel more tired and low on energy than usual. Try some calming meditations that help you relax and connect with the earth.

Focus on feeling the ground beneath you, under your feet or pelvis, and let go of any tension with each exhale. Imagine sinking deeper into the earth, feeling supported and at peace. Reflect on the grounding and calming effects of these meditations and incorporate them into your self-care routine.

Phase 2: Follicular

Now it's time to nourish our body. Feel the support of the ground beneath you and draw nourishment from the earth. Inhale deeply, bringing nourishment to your womb and any areas that need it, and exhale any tension. Focus on feeling connected and at peace, letting your body and mind relax. Reflect on the activities or habits that make you feel most nourished and at peace and incorporate them into your daily routine. Consider writing down a few nourishing activities you can engage in during this phase and try to include them in your schedule.

Phase 3: Ovulation

During this active phase, focus on creating space and warmth within yourself. Imagine each breath expanding and softening your body, like a river flowing freely. Picture a wide, open sky and feel the warmth of the sun radiating onto you, recharging your body with each breath. Reflect on the activities or interactions that bring you the most joy and energy during this phase. Write down your top three energizing activities and make an effort to incorporate them into your life during this phase.

Phase 4: Luteal

In this phase, aim for lightness, ease, and self-compassion. Let your spine rise effortlessly, like a tree growing from the earth. With each inhale, feel your heart lifting toward the sky and imagine a gentle smile spreading across your face. Send this inner smile to your womb with each exhale, welcoming whatever comes your way with kindness and self-care. Reflect on how you can practice self-compassion and kindness toward yourself. Make a list of self-care activities that help you feel nurtured and supported and choose one or two to focus on during this phase.

Integrating Rhythm in Relationships

Communication Strategies

Haven't we all had an argument with either our partner or a work colleague during our period? It happens! But here's the thing: Effective communication can make a significant difference in maintaining strong relationships, whether personal or professional. Reflect on the ways in which you can communicate your needs and feelings during this time, and practice expressing yourself openly and kindly.

Menstrual cycles can mess with our hormones and energy levels, which causes mood shifts, affecting everything from chores to social plans. It's important to be open with those around us about how we're feeling, especially when we're dealing with PMS symptoms like cramps or mood swings or if our libido changes.

Communication is more than just talking; it's also about understanding ourselves better and helping our partners and coworkers do the same. The more we embody our truth, the more confidence we will have during these conversations—and the more confidence we have, the better able we are to express ourselves in the best possible way to convey our message during these times. It's empowering to share with and guide our partners and colleagues to help them understand what we're going through. We can encourage them to ask questions or just be present with us, as their presence will help us as women feel supported and safe. After all, sharing how we feel and explaining our state of mind can clear up misunderstandings and release stress.

Support Networks

Most of us women bleed every month, and some of us face health issues and challenges related to our cycle, but these issues often remain hidden due to stigma and silence. To address this, we need open dialogue and support from our friends, family, colleagues, and wider community to normalize menstruation and its impact on our day-to-day lives. Reflect on how you can foster such open dialogue in your own circles and consider initiating conversations to break the stigma.

Educating young girls not only about menstrual health but also about the shifts in their mood can empower them to manage their symptoms, identify disorders, and prioritize self-care, ultimately reducing stigma and promoting inclusivity and sustainability. The community we seek can start with ourselves. We can start with our friends, sisters, mothers, aunts, cousins, and even our own daughters. Whether you are a man or a woman reading this, it is our collective responsibility to share what we know and provide what we seek to others to allow us all to grow together. This is the most real thing in life.

Case Studies and Success Stories

Real-Life Examples

Melanie, a 45-year-old software developer, shares her story of adjusting her routine to sync with her monthly cycle. Reflect on Melanie's experience and consider how you can apply similar strategies to your own life. Think about ways in which you can adjust your routine to better align with your cycle and improve your overall well-being:

"I've had severe PCOS for more than 15 years, and it's gotten worse over time. Dealing with my menstrual cycle has been tough. Around ovulation, I have intense pain for a day, making it hard to move. The week before my period, I feel terrible. But when my period comes, it's a relief because I feel normal again.

"Dealing with this every month is tough. Previously, I had a less flexible job, and it was much harder. I had mood swings and I felt my partner didn't understand me. On his part, he thought I was moody for no reason. We almost broke up, but with the help of a friend we talked things out, understood the gap in communication, and worked on it. I switched jobs and now have flexible work arrangements, and I no longer let my frustration due to a tough work routine near ovulation spoil my relationship. With my partner's support, I have stayed productive, and he now understands that on some days I need space and silent support."

Cynthia, a teacher in her late 20s, has this to say:

"For the past five months, I've been diligently tracking my menstrual cycle in a graph-ruled notebook. Each day, I jot down a sentence about how I feel, creating a detailed record of my emotional and physiological patterns. Over time, this data has become a valuable tool for predicting my mood and energy levels, as well as my periods.

"I've noticed that toward the end of my cycle, during the luteal phase, my social energy dips significantly. So, I've learned to adjust my social calendar and commitments accordingly. By managing my schedule in this way, I can prioritize self-care and be fully present with friends when I do spend time with them."

Lessons Learned

From the anecdotes I've just shared above, it's clear that we can empower ourselves by aligning with our hormonal patterns instead of trying to manipulate them by using medicines. By listening to our bodies and embracing cyclical self-care, we can find balance and grace in our lives.

Cynthia's experience of "cycle syncing," using her moods and body signals to guide her daily activities, is encouraging. This approach goes beyond traditional hormone tracking, as it involves lifestyle adjustment around her cycle. With the rise of period-tracking apps, syncing with our cycle has become more accessible.

Melanie's story shows how important it is to communicate with our significant other to help them understand if we have problems during certain days of our cycle. It also shows that we have to make workplace adjustments by asking for either period leave or a work-from-home option.

The bottom line is that our period is not an isolated event; there is a cycle involved, so we have to let the rhythm of our body guide our routine.

To Conclude: Moving Forward in Harmony

It's important to know that having a period is normal, healthy, and empowering. Embracing our period with positivity as a reminder of our womanhood and our connection to creation can help us understand our body better. By learning the different tools we need in each phase, we can feel good throughout our cycle and ensure we always have variety in our life.

It's not just about dealing with periods; it's about respecting our body's wisdom and enjoying its unique rhythm. By adjusting our lifestyle to match our menstrual cycle, we can use our body's natural wisdom to improve our lives. Ways to sync our life with our cycle include:

- **Cycle-syncing foods:** Using a chart to choose foods that match each phase of our cycle to give our body what it needs.

- **Exercise based on our cycle:** Changing our workouts depending on where we are in our cycle—for example, choosing gentle exercises during our period and increasing the intensity as we get closer to ovulation.

- **Meditation, yoga and mindfulness:** Using appropriate mindfulness techniques for each phase of our cycle to become more one with ourselves and live in harmony with life.

Call to Action

- Ready to sync your life with your body's rhythms? Start small and deepen your connection with your body. Experiment, and let your body lead.

- Track your cycle using apps like Flo or Clue. Pay attention to changes and listen to your body.

- Track your cycle length, symptoms, energy, sleep, and sex drive.

- Adjust your diet and exercise to support your cycle.

- Embrace the ebb and flow, whether it's a massage during your period or outdoor activities in the follicular phase.

Chapter 4:
Emotional Landscapes

Our emotional landscape is created by the usual range of feelings we experience and it's where we feel most comfortable. It's like our emotional home base. The ups and downs of our menstrual cycle are key in shaping our emotional landscape. In this chapter, we explore how periods and emotional well-being are connected, focusing on the roller coaster of emotions many of us go through during our menstrual cycle. This journey aims to uncover the subtle ways in which our cycle impacts our emotions, giving all women the tools to handle these changes with insight and kindness.

Embracing Our Inner Seasons

Throughout our monthly cycle, our body goes through regular changes in mood and energy due to our hormones. Like a beautiful symphony of changing hormones, our cycle guides how we feel emotionally, how strong we are, and how we express ourselves.

Estrogen, which rises at certain times, can make us feel happier and more alert. But when progesterone drops suddenly before our period, it might cause mood swings. I personally feel my most dramatic in the last three days of my cycle. It takes a lot of effort to bring myself to a balance, and I find so many reasons to cry.

The way our menstrual cycle affects mood isn't just about hormones; our feelings are also influenced by psychological and sociocultural factors. The way we see our bodies and society's attitudes toward periods also play a big role. To feel better overall, and to have emotional balance, it's important to understand our inner movements, plan our life based on our cycle, and take care of our overall well-being. This could range from eating omega-3-rich foods, exercising frequently, and cultivating mindfulness to engaging in activities like meditation.

Aside from the physical and cultural aspects, there's also a spiritual dimension to our periods. Our inner goddess—the powerhouse of our femininity—holds deep emotions and wisdom in our bodies. It's a space for both life and death, a channel for creativity and birth, symbolized by the flow of blood. Sadly, many women don't realize the sacredness of their own blood and, unfortunately, perceive it as dirty.

The goal of this chapter is to empower our inner goddess. By understanding and managing our emotions through the perspective of female archetypes and menstrual phases, we can tap into our inner strength and wisdom.

Spring–The Maiden (Post-Menstruation)

My first period came as a surprise, but my mother's gentle guidance turned it into a celebration of womanhood. She taught me to honor this phase as a time of new beginnings and self-discovery. –Darya

New Beginnings and Renewal

Archetypes, representing different aspects of our psyche, provide a powerful way to connect with our menstrual cycle, offering traits and attitudes that allow us to achieve balance. The Maiden (sometimes known as the Rebel) archetype symbolizes the inner spring, occurring between our period and ovulation. Similar to our teenage years or when menstruation begins, this phase signifies renewal, fresh starts, and energy. Hormone levels rise, especially estradiol, boosting motivation.

The Maiden represents youth, beauty, and the excitement of new beginnings. She's in the process of discovering herself, embracing her sexuality, and finding her balance. Fun, flirty, and carefree, yet focused and determined, she embodies the feelings and emotions mirrored in the cycles of our bodies, the earth, and the moon. As women, we are connected to this energy—and it can be easy to get stuck in it, always seeking novelty and youthfulness. However, embracing Maiden energy can sometimes be beneficial, especially when embarking on new adventures or challenges in life, whether it's traveling, starting a business, or changing direction.

The Maiden symbolizes youth. As we often explore, experiment, establish our identities, and push boundaries in youth, in a way we are embodying the Rebel spirit within us. This phase encourages risk-taking and forging our own paths, whether it's trying out unconventional hairstyles, relationships, or adventures. The Maiden phase is more about a mindset than whether someone is sexually active.

The Maiden is often portrayed as unmarried, self-sufficient, pure, and strong-willed. She emerges when women start prioritizing their own desires and goals. She's full of energy, smart, down-to-earth, and brimming with confidence, effortlessly balancing work and life.

In the past, when women were expected to prioritize caring for others, the Maiden was sometimes viewed as selfish. But as society evolves and women worldwide pursue their dreams, the Maiden is making a comeback. She's being embraced and celebrated, highlighting that life isn't just about marriage and motherhood anymore.

Have you ever connected with your inner Maiden? She's there, waiting to emerge, but you might need to adjust your approach to meet your own needs and desires.

Strategies for the Maiden

Reconnect with your Maiden self by reflecting on your teen and young adult years. Remember the music you loved, the movies you watched, and your Hollywood crushes. Create a playlist of your favorite songs from that time and listen to it while engaging in an activity that brings you joy. While you don't have to return to that style, browsing old photos or keepsakes can help you reconnect with your past self. Consider creating a collage as a creative exercise. Bring the vibrance you once held, the excitement you once had, back to your life today, using the dynamism in your body as an imprint.

You should also make time for play! Schedule a "play date" with yourself or with friends, where you engage in fun activities like board games, dancing, or creative arts.

Try something new! As the energy of this period is represented by spring, it's a perfect time to plant a new seed and start something new. Whether it's a class, hobby, hairstyle, or lipstick shade, embrace novelty. Write down three new activities you've always wanted to try and pick one to start this week. Both the Rebel and the Maiden encourage doing things because they feel good, regardless of others' opinions. Don't limit yourself when it comes to reading, watching, or listening to anything that will inspire and drive you.

Plan ahead! Whether it's your next holiday, a work project, your wedding, or simply organizing your schedule, tapping into the Maiden's energy involves strategy and planning. So, whenever you engage in these activities, you're connecting with her energy. Be yourself and embrace your personality.

Dress in a way that boosts your confidence, whether it's killer heels or comfy yoga pants. Strengthen your self-esteem by focusing on your solar plexus chakra, and consider using essential oils like frankincense and rose for clarity and confidence. Remember to prioritize rest to prevent burnout, especially during high-energy phases.

Apt Description

Reawakened, rejuvenated, clean slate, new beginning, dynamic and energetic, attentive, adventurous.

Summer—The Mother (Ovulatory Phase)

During my ovulation phase, I feel like I can conquer the world. It's when I feel most connected to my creativity and my desire to nurture those around me. –Ani

Nurturing Growth and Connection

Summer marks the beginning of ovulation. This phase is our peak fertility time. Hormone levels soar, thickening our womb lining for potential pregnancy. Energy levels skyrocket and we feel extra charismatic, putting more effort into our appearance. Confidence, high self-esteem, and a boosted libido are common during this "menstrual summer." Our communication skills shine, making social interactions smoother—perfect for a first date.

Since you're super fertile, it's important to double-check your birth control if pregnancy isn't in your plans (in which case, you should be doing this regularly anyway!). Opt for a low-carb, high-fiber diet. Exercise feels particularly gratifying during this phase, empowering you to tackle anything that comes your way!

Our Mother archetype also shines brightest during this ovulatory phase, which is a time of high energy. Identify a project or relationship that needs nurturing and devote time to it, ensuring you channel your abundant energy into something meaningful.

The Mother embodies not just birthing and nurturing but also strength, wisdom, and a deep connection to nature. Plan a nature walk or gardening session to connect with the earth and reflect on your nurturing qualities. The Mother's nurturing energy encourages us to blossom in our own path, promoting growth rather than control.

Central to her essence is presence, care, and attention. Through her, we learn to nurture our creations, whether they are children, projects, or ideas, and to safeguard our environment and ourselves. She grants us clarity, allowing us to see ourselves and our lives without bias.

When our inner Mother thrives, we feel compelled to care for our mind, body, and soul, recognizing that self-care is vital for positive change. However, it's necessary to channel her energy wisely, avoiding both suppression and burnout.

Living as the Mother

The summer phase brings both literal and metaphorical heat into our lives as ovulation kicks in.

During the Mother phase, our energy becomes more outward and expressive. We feel extra social, making it a prime time for community engagement, nurturing relationships, and lending a helping hand through hosting, cooking, or other acts of service.

To nurture your Mother archetype, these simple steps are helpful: Slow down and appreciate the present; simplify your life by focusing on what truly matters without being side-tracked; let go of perfectionism (you are already good enough); incorporate a simple ritual like journaling or celebrating the moon cycles; be resourceful and seek support when needed; and learn new practical skills to challenge yourself, as the Mother is very resourceful. Connect with nature through gardening or outdoor activities; work on emotional balance by strengthening your heart chakra and practicing unconditional love; tune into your menstrual cycle and align with the natural rhythms of the world; and, finally, wear comfortable clothes that allow you to move freely.

Apt Description

Flirtatious, lively, outgoing and sociable, helpful, bridge-builder, supportive, nonjudgmental, nurturer and carer.

Autumn—The Witch (Pre-Menstruation)

The luteal phase brings a whirlwind of emotions, but I've learned to embrace it as a time for deep reflection and honest self-expression. It's my time to confront my inner truths. –Sarah

Reflection and Self-Focus

During the autumn of our cycle, also known as the luteal phase, our body is trying to figure out if it needs to get ready for a baby. When there is no baby, our progesterone levels, which were super high beforehand, start to drop.

At the start of our menstrual autumn, things might not seem too bad. We might feel chill and relaxed, and sleep like a rock. But as progesterone decreases, we might start feeling down. It's like a blue mood takes over. Concentrating becomes a challenge, and we might have to deal with headaches, tender breasts, mood swings, sugar cravings, queasiness, and skin issues.

Here's the thing: Society hasn't quite caught up to how people feel in the week leading up to their period. So, we sometimes feel pretty alone and misunderstood. Our emotions during this time can be all over the place: One minute, we're craving cuddles on the couch, and the next, we just want to curl up and cry. It's important to be kind to ourselves during this phase.

It's a good time to add more vitamin B, magnesium, and calcium to our diet to support our body, as these nutrients are important for blood production. Foods such as lentils, liver, and bone broth are excellent choices. Additionally, consider easing up on intense workouts. Instead, try a gentle yoga session or a relaxing walk to help ground yourself. Your body and mind will benefit from the change.

Our Witch archetype makes an appearance in the autumn of our cycle. During this time, we're not as lively as before. Instead, we're more contemplative, focusing on ourselves, our needs, and our harvests.

Think of the Witch in old stories who was often feared. Similarly, many of us dread our inner Witch because this phase can be challenging. It's like a dark side of ourselves. Our inner Witch craves solitude and might even push people away in a not-so-friendly manner without us realizing it. Set aside "me time" for solitude and reflection. Consider a digital detox or a day spent in nature to recharge.

But the Witch makes up for all this trouble by being a healer. She's like the wise woman within us who understands that we can't keep moving forward without taking breaks to reflect and process all that we've experienced. She knows that true healing isn't just about covering up wounds and soldiering on; it's about digging deep to address the root cause.

Harnessing the Witch's Power

So, how do we make friends with our inner Witch? It's all about tuning in to our body's signals and treating ourselves with love and kindness. When we disregard these signals, they often become louder, resulting in heightened irritability and fatigue, among other issues.

Listening closely to what our body needs and responding with care is the key to embracing our inner Witch. It's better to draw inward, find more space and solitude, and ignore the pileup of demands. Create a peaceful space at home with calming elements like candles and soft music, and spend time there daily for reflection and relaxation.

As an entrepreneur, I align my sessions, classes, and commitments with my cycle, deliberately planning downtime before it begins to prioritize my well-being. I bring the following advice to the attention of every woman I work with, and now to the wider world in this book: Before menstruation, spend time alone in reflection. This is a precious time for us, as it can lead to creative inspiration. This can begin with creating a peaceful spot in our homes, such as a small altar dedicated to our feminine energy and personal growth, adorned with fresh flowers, candles, a water fountain, crystals, and pleasant scents.

We can also make space for ourselves by engaging in a digital detox, at least overnight, and having the courage to cancel some of our calendar obligations, prioritizing ourselves. It's essential to learn to set boundaries and not just take action because someone else demands it.

Deciding to honor this inner journey of winding down takes courage and self-love. It takes time to turn these practices into a muscle that becomes organic. When we embrace our body's cues during the autumn or Witch phase (also know as the Wild Woman or Priestess phase), we might feel as if we're overflowing with inspiration, eager to channel our waning energy into creative pursuits. It's the perfect moment to nurture personal insights, pen poetry, sketch, brainstorm business or career strategies, and assert our identity. It's also the perfect time to work on developing our throat chakra because we are learning to have a voice, to raise our voice, and to share our needs. This is directly related to surrendering, which enables us to accept our obligations, let go of what no longer serves us, and practice speaking our truth. Additionally, it's a great time to learn abdominal massage—there are many videos on YouTube—for comforting our womb and preparing for the upcoming phase. A hot magnesium bath or a natural face mask can also help to nurture and nourish both our inner woman and our body.

Apt Description

Imaginative, temperamental, disordered and awkward, lazy and inactive, more innovative and full of ideas, ambitious, tactical but easily distracted.

Winter—The Wise Woman (Menstruation)

Menstruation used to be my least favorite time of the month, but now I see it as a sacred pause. It's when I gather my strength, reflect on my journey, and plan for the future. –Kristina

Think of our period like the winter season for our body, when we feel more emotional and tired and experience common symptoms like back pain, bloating, and cramps. Just like in nature, winter is the time to reflect, and we should use this phase to contemplate how we want our next cycle to be based on the lessons we received from the previous cycle.

Through our menstrual winter, we sometimes notice mood swings or feel a bit cranky. It's common to struggle with negative thoughts throughout this time. We are naturally inclined to take it easy over the first few days of our period, giving ourselves some extra rest and care. Remembering that bleeding is a ceremony on a spiritual level, and very hard work on a physical level, we need to make the time and space for ourselves to allow the natural flow to happen and energies to align.

Just like winter, the bleeding phase of our cycle is a time to rest and take care of ourselves. It's okay to slow down, recharge, and connect with our blood, remembering how rich it is, how sacred it is, and how much creative power and how many dreams it holds. Focus on eating iron-rich foods and staying hydrated instead of giving in to sugar cravings. Dark chocolate, with its magnesium content, can help soothe cramps and boost mood.

For those of us who do not bleed, we still carry the creative energy of womanhood. Whether you're in menopause or struggling with infertility, you're connected to the wisdom of womanhood in your own unique way. Remember, in shamanism and many ancient cultures, women are considered wise when they are free from their period. In most tribes in the Amazonian jungle, women can become *curanderas* and hold space in ceremonies only after they have reached menopause. Let's remember to celebrate every phase of our life.

Guidance From the Wise Woman

Winter is a time for looking inside ourselves and changing in a special way. When we are in our winter phase, we might feel annoyed if people ask us to do things for them. Winter is about taking care of ourselves, not just giving to others. Create a self-care routine for your menstruation days, including activities like warm baths, gentle yoga, and journaling about your feelings and insights. It's important to be kind to ourselves during this time, for our own happiness and for our families. Practice self-compassion by writing down positive affirmations and reading them daily. Share your experiences and wisdom with close friends or a support group. Personally, I enjoy taking baths, watching movies with my partner, spending quiet time alone writing or reading in bed, sleeping, and being outside in nature. I do my best not to resist change; instead, I move with the flow. After all, the Wise Woman is the queen of metamorphosis. While she may appear frightening at first, she will guide us to rebirth and rejuvenation

But there's more to it than just resting our bodies; there is also something magical about this phase. Long ago, wise women believed that during the winter phase, the line between our world and the spirit world gets thinner. Women on their period were thought to be extra powerful and wise. In ancient times, women would go to special places during their period to connect with the spirit world and renew themselves. Nowadays, we can turn to meditation and writing to help us think deeply during this time. Let's value our own experiences and share our insights with others without imposing our beliefs on them. Practice self-love by looking into the mirror and exploring the depths of what you see in yourself. Accept yourself completely, including your physical appearance and any changes, during this phase, allowing your intuition to guide you freely.

Apt Description

Solitude, peace, space, sensitivity, alone time, rest, rejuvenation, intuitiveness, creativity, loosening up.

Conclusion: Integrating Our Emotional Cycle

The link between our menstrual cycle and our emotions reveals how complex our bodies are, showing the deep connection between our physical and mental well-being. Understanding this connection allows us women to navigate our emotional ups and downs with more awareness and kindness, leading to a sense of empowerment and overall wellness.

By paying attention to our energetic patterns, we can deepen our connection to our womanhood and gain insight into our own cycles. This awareness helps us understand ourselves better and recognize when something feels off.

Let's welcome these archetypes in our cycle, reflecting changes in our energy and behavioral patterns. Let's accept each phase as an opportunity for personal development, helping us overcome obstacles. Let's prioritize our own needs and well-being.

Call to Action

- Embrace the cyclical nature of emotions during your menstrual cycle.

- Let's commit to understanding and practicing self-care techniques that support us through every phase.

- Let's cultivate resilience, self-compassion, and empowerment. On airplanes, we're always asked to put on our own oxygen masks before assisting loved ones. Taking care of ourselves enables us to provide better care for the people around us.

Chapter 5: Grandmother Power (Ancient Wisdom)

Tapping Into Ancestral Wisdom

Ancient wisdom, often referred to as grandmother wisdom, is a treasure trove of knowledge passed down through generations. It's the wisdom our ancestors gained from living closely with nature and each other, but sadly, it's often overlooked by modern science. Take a moment to reflect on the wisdom passed down in your family. Write down a piece of advice or a tradition that has been shared with you.

This wisdom holds beliefs and values guiding how we care for our world, along with traditions for living harmoniously with nature. It also includes the practical knowledge gained from our own experiences.

Our womb, a sacred library, holds incredible grandmother wisdom waiting to be unlocked. As women, we're connected to nature's rhythm through our "moon time" (periods).

In this chapter, we explore our ancestral wisdom, rediscovering women's ancient healing and living practices. Let's journey back in time and tap into the wisdom of our ancestors together.

Wisdom Across Cultures

Like diverse ecosystems in nature, cultures bloom with their own customs, traditions, and perspectives regarding our monthly cycle, each adding its own vibrant hue to the tapestry of human experience. In the hunter-gatherer societies of our early human ancestors, women's periods were seen positively, with no feelings of being dirty.

Even today, in some traditional societies, menstrual rituals help women feel safe and strong. So, being isolated during menstruation can be seen either as being pushed away for being impure or as a chance to take a break from chores and recharge. In some places, our period is seen as something to hide, while in others, it's celebrated without any shame.

Many traditional communities believe that menstruation should align with the natural rhythms of the universe. This idea is deeply rooted in their myths and rituals. French anthropologist Claude Lévi-Strauss studied these myths and concluded that they reflect a concern about the chaos that might result if women's periods were not synchronized with the universe (Waldorf & Grollemond, 2024).

In some ancient cultures, women on their period were seen as special and strong. They were believed to have extra psychic powers and could even heal the sick. Some stories say that if a menstruating woman walks naked in a field, bugs fall off the corn, showing her power. Menstrual blood was thought to be dangerous to men's strength. In Africa, it was used in powerful magic spells for both good and bad purposes.

In Aboriginal Australia, there's a belief that synchronized cycles bring spiritual power and fertility, represented by the "Rainbow Snake." And in Mayan mythology, menstrual blood is believed to turn into creatures used in sorcery before the moon goddess is reborn from it.

In cultures where women's blood is seen as sacred, it's believed to have special powers. An Indian artist named Lyla FreeChild used her menstrual blood to paint a picture of a powerful goddess she saw in a dream. She believes menstrual blood has creative and healing powers (Waldorf & Grollemond, 2024).

Sociologist Emile Durkheim proposed that religion emerged from the menstruation phenomenon, where the sight of blood created a symbolic separation between men and women. In ancient societies, blood was often associated with fear and taboo. Thus, rituals were designed to dispel these fears and taboos; these rituals took the shape of early religious rituals and practices (Waldorf & Grollemond, 2024).

In different parts of the world, there are unique traditions around menstruation:

● In Zambia, women use a cloth called a *chitenge* to catch menstrual blood. When girls have their first period, it's seen as a sign that they're ready for adult responsibilities. Older women then teach them about sex, marriage, and how to manage menstruation, but it's taboo to talk about periods with men.

● In parts of South Asia, there's a taboo around menstruation, with many considering it impure. Girls may face restrictions on what they can do and eat during their period, and some even miss school because of it.

● In India, menarche, or a girl's first period, is celebrated. In places like Andhra Pradesh, girls receive gifts and celebrations to mark this important milestone.

● In the Tulu Nadu region of Karnataka, South India, there's a festival called Keddaso, or "Menstruation of Mother Earth." It's believed that Mother Earth menstruates, and the festival celebrates this idea.

● In Sumba, Indonesia, women keep their menstrual cycles secret, believing it gives them power over men. They think that by keeping secrets, they can control more than they actually can.

● In Ivory Coast, periods are compared to the flower of a tree and are believed to be necessary, just like the flower is needed before the tree can bear fruit (Waldorf & Grollemond, 2024).

Think about the rituals you practice or would like to introduce during your menstrual cycle. How could these rituals help you feel more connected and empowered?

Common Themes and Lessons

Different cultures hold varying beliefs and practices regarding periods. Broadly, these beliefs fall into two contrasting perspectives: Some cultures regard the monthly cycle as a normal and empowering aspect of growing up, while others think of it as dirty, impure, and shameful, leading to secrecy and concealment. For instance, women in India and Nepal may feel embarrassed and hide their moon time from men, while in Ghana, girls entering puberty are celebrated with special ceremonies and gifts.

These differing viewpoints fit with the grandmother wisdom shared in these cultures. The rituals and ceremonies associated with periods are centered around respecting nature, coming together as a community, and connecting spiritually. Consider creating a small ceremony or ritual to honor your menstrual cycle. This could include lighting a candle, meditating, or journaling about your experiences and feelings. It's about living in harmony with the environment and celebrating the earth, plants, and animals. It also highlights the importance of supporting each other and finding strength in unity. Spiritual practices, like prayer and meditation, help us navigate life's challenges and connect with something greater than ourselves.

Practical Teachings and Their Applications

Health and Healing

We've not only studied how ancient cultures used natural resources for staying healthy, but we've also explored traditional community health practices to find solutions for modern illnesses. Through the wisdom passed down by grandmothers, we find traditional ways to help with periods. These include simple things like herbal teas and using hot water bottles to ease discomfort and help us feel better overall. Grandmothers might also suggest eating more foods with iron to stay healthy during menstruation, or creating a meal plan that includes iron-rich foods during our menstrual cycle. These old-school remedies can work alongside modern medicine, giving us holistic solutions for both our body and mind. While modern treatments are helpful, adding in traditional remedies can give us extra support and keep us connected to our cultural roots. Plus, using these age-old practices makes us feel empowered and in control of our own health.

For centuries, different cultures have used traditional medicines to help women with their health and gynecological issues. People who work with these remedies have learned a lot over time and have come up with many effective treatments. This knowledge has been passed down and improved upon through modern science and medicine. Many things can affect how we experience periods, like what we eat, how we live, and our cultural beliefs. Modern medicine has learned a lot from traditional practices, using what nature has given us to treat illnesses and help people feel better, no matter where they come from. A case in point is how some traditional medicines are relevant in modern times, with these practices vouched for by modern research. Consider the following examples:

- In traditional Chinese medicine (TCM), menstruation is called "heavenly water." Emotional stress is believed to directly impact the monthly cycle. When a woman has her period, the advice is to keep warm and avoid cold foods, opting for warm, cooked meals like soups instead. Rest is important, as is reducing stress and avoiding sex. Inverted yoga poses are encouraged for downward blood flow. After a woman's period, nourishing the blood with foods like beef, liver, and dark leafy greens is recommended, whereas before her period, the focus is on relieving tension with gentle exercise and relaxation techniques like qigong and yoga.

- In Ayurveda, simple practices are believed to promote menstrual health and overall well-being. Eating warm, cooked meals that contain spices like ginger and cinnamon aids in cleansing. Rest is encouraged, as is avoiding activities that disrupt downward energy flow to support the body's natural processes. Reflecting and staying hydrated with warm teas are also beneficial. Other Ayurvedic practices include seasonal cleansing, maintaining a daily routine, self-massage, regular exercise, and practicing pranayama and yoga.

Relationships and Community Building

To maintain strong family ties and build community, elders advise embracing family traditions that convey our values and beliefs, promoting a sense of identity and belonging. These traditions ground us in our culture and shape our interactions with the world from birth, providing stability, love, and emotional support. Family dynamics influence our personal development, offering encouragement and belonging as we face life's challenges. Strong emotional ties foster security and reduce feelings of loneliness. Sharing family stories daily not only connects younger generations to their heritage but also brings joy to the storyteller by recalling cherished memories.

Elders stress the importance of maintaining connections to enhance their well-being and community ties. Communication with elders is more than social; it's imperative for their support network and personal identity. Senior bonding enriches the entire family, preserving family history and wisdom for future generations.

Indigenous communities offer the best example of how strong family relationships and friendships are essential not just for community building but for growing old well. Their communities are all about living according to cultural values like honesty and treating others with respect. Collective well-being is a priority, with children seen as precious gifts meant to strengthen bonds and care for one another. Families often live together and share childcare responsibilities, with everyone feeling responsible for both their own family and all children in the community. Elders play a central role in passing down cultural knowledge and traditions, emphasizing living in harmony with the environment and showing love, respect, and compassion for others. Intergenerational connections are highly valued, as they ensure the preservation of cultural values and traditions for future generations (Burke, 2023).

Practical Advice on Improving Relationships Based on Respect, Empathy, and Support

Improving relationships centers around the fundamental principles of respect, empathy, and support. In the journey of relationships, challenges often arise like unexpected storms, but facing them head-on is key. Discussing rough patches, addressing misunderstandings promptly, and remaining open to different perspectives can help smooth out the bumps. Open lines of communication, where all family members feel heard and respected, strengthen family bonds. Actively listening to each other is important, as is giving each other our full attention and committing to healthy relationships through solid social networks and effective communication. Offering support and encouragement during challenging times, and celebrating each other's successes, nurtures a sense of partnership and mutual respect.

Barriers, whether physical, emotional, or perceptual, can hold back connection. Recognizing these walls and finding gentle ways to connect is vital. For seniors, encouraging strong family relationships offers comfort and emotional support, enhancing happiness and well-being. Engaging in community activities provides a sense of purpose and belonging, promoting healthy aging. Empathy, the ability to appreciate and respond to others' feelings, plays a pivotal role in relationship dynamics.

Empathy allows us to step into another's shoes, nurturing emotional connection and improving communication. By understanding each other's perspective, we can address underlying issues, reduce conflict, and promote mutual respect. Empathy enriches relationships by cultivating emotional bonds, enhancing communication, and promoting effective conflict resolution. Cultivating empathy can lead to deeper, more meaningful connections in all relationships.

Identify a family tradition that you cherish or would like to start. Share it with your family and friends, and explore how it strengthens your connections.

Spiritual Connections and Rituals—Spiritual Practices Passed Down

Grandmothers have long passed down spiritual rituals surrounding menstruation, offering insights into connecting with oneself and the universe. Across cultures, menstruation was once viewed as a time of heightened spiritual and mental power for women. Ancient traditions, like those of the Egyptians and Greeks, incorporated menstrual blood into rituals for spiritual empowerment and fertility. In Hawaiian and Celtic cultures, menstruation was considered a sacred time, symbolizing spiritual strength and connection to the divine.

Elder women in Celtic Britain were revered for their wisdom, which was believed to be heightened by their postmenopausal state. Rituals involving menstrual blood, like staining graves or seclusion, symbolized a deep connection to the earth and the divine feminine. The practice of secluding menstruating women reflects a reverence for their power and the need for inward reflection.

The menstrual cycle itself is seen as a ritual, fostering deeper connection and self-healing. These sacred rituals go beyond self-care, awakening a sense of reverence and self-love. By embracing these practices, we can rewire our brains and bodies to embrace the beauty and power of the feminine cycle (Waldorf & Grollemond, 2024).

Try incorporating a spiritual ritual into your menstrual cycle, such as a moon meditation or a nature walk. Observe how this enhances your connection with yourself and the world around you.

Integrating Ancient Rituals Today

Crafting a special ceremony for our menstrual cycle is a wonderful way to honor our body's rhythms, listen to our needs, and connect with our inner wisdom. Create a personal ritual that celebrates your menstrual cycle. This could involve elements like music, dance, or art. Reflect on how this practice deepens your connection to your body and its natural rhythms. Embracing the sacredness of our moon time not only heals us but also contributes to the healing of our ancestors, society, and future generations. Reclaiming this sacred time transforms it from a perceived curse into a profound blessing for the world. By acknowledging and respecting the discomfort and challenges of our period, we tap into ancestral pain and open ourselves to a deeper connection with Mother Earth and the cycles of creation. You're welcome to explore these rituals, share them, and engage in the discussion.

Returning our blood to the earth in a deliberate manner is a sacred act of reciprocity with our original Mother, linking womb to womb. It's a way of expressing gratitude for all that the earth provides us and acknowledging our interconnection. Using a menstrual cup makes this process simple, allowing us to release our blood into nature, whether in a garden or in the wilderness.

Similarly, offering our blood to bodies of water, particularly the vast expanse of the ocean, is a way to honor the feminine essence of water. This act, reminiscent of mermaid rituals, celebrates our emotional and lunar selves. We can either use a menstrual cup while swimming or allow ourselves to bleed freely into the water, accompanied by prayers or blessings.

Lying under the moon or the night sky during menstruation is essential for reconnecting with the yin aspects of life, which are often overlooked in our fast-paced world. This practice, known as moon bathing, helps us embrace the magic and medicine of the night. Consistent moon bathing can even help regulate our menstrual cycle, as it aligns us with the rhythms of the moon (Willemaine-Green, 2020).

Stories of Resilience and Strength—Inspirational Anecdotes

Marisol Kiyoko and Resilience

Sometimes, an unassuming demeanor and a quiet personality hide an incredibly brave person who has the most remarkable stories to tell. Marisol Kiyoko Guevara exemplified this; her composure hints at nothing of her extraordinary journey. With a gentle smile, she speaks of overcoming abuse, life-threatening situations, and societal stereotypes. Her modesty and genuine laughter reveal a woman of incredible resilience.

Marisol faced literal and metaphorical mountains in her life, from surviving perilous situations in the Himalayas to being abandoned by her father at a young age. Raised by her single mother, she learned the power of perseverance and determination.

Her courage inspired her to leave an abusive marriage, despite feeling worthless and fearful. She embarked on a journey of self-discovery, traveling to over 40 countries and overcoming challenges like trekking the Annapurna circuit with a failing knee and confronting aggressive guard dogs.

Through her experiences, Marisol learned the importance of resilience and determination. She encourages women to speak up, seek support, and pursue their goals fearlessly. As a chess champion turned successful entrepreneur, she sees life as a strategic game where we must be bold and assertive. She calls for men to be allies by investing in female-led businesses and supporting women's voices.

Marisol's story reminds us that quiet strength and resilience can lead to extraordinary accomplishments, and that asking for help is a sign of courage, not weakness (Resende, 2023).

Reflect on a challenging experience in your life when you demonstrated resilience. Write about how you overcame the obstacles and what you learned from the experience. Share your story with others to inspire and empower them.

Chrys Nguyen's Story of Providing Community Care and Support

Chrys is a member of "Sisters of Providence," providing healthcare to communities in Alaska. Born in Vietnam, when she was an infant she fled with her family on a boat. She was raised with a deep appreciation for community service and exposure to diverse beliefs, and her parents instilled in her the importance of independence and compassion. They taught her to prioritize self-care and emotional well-being—essential lessons that shaped her approach to caregiving.

Chrys emphasizes the significance of processing emotions and finding solutions to overcome challenges. Grounded in her upbringing, she continues her family's tradition of social accountability, passing down values of gratitude and community support to her own children. In Asian culture, the concept of family extends beyond nuclear relatives to encompass the broader community, a principle Chrys embraces wholeheartedly.

Her commitment to community is echoed in her unconventional approach to parenting, which emphasizes the importance of collective care and support (Providence Health Team, n.d.).

Conclusion: Embracing the Grandmother Spirit

Unlocking the grandmother spirit means tapping into ancient wisdom for personal growth and insight. Forget the usual textbooks; let's explore our inner truths. Identify a piece of ancient wisdom that resonates with you and think about how you can apply it to your daily life. Share this wisdom with someone close to you and discuss its impact.

By learning from ancient knowledge, we can make sense of life's twists and turns, discovering a purpose behind every encounter and experience.

Though some have tried to hide this wisdom, it's still out there for the curious. Even science is starting to see the value in ancient teachings. Our life isn't just random; it's like a story with a plan, but we still have the freedom to choose our own adventure along the way.

Moving Forward With Ancient Insights

Embracing the wisdom of the ages and weaving it into our daily lives helps create a bridge between past and present. Make a list of three ancient practices or pieces of wisdom that you find valuable. Plan how you can incorporate these practices into your routine and observe the changes they bring to your life.

The journey of our present is one of evolution, adaptation, and progress, all rooted in the teachings of the past. Rather than seeing past wisdom as a prison, let's recognize it as a valuable teacher, guiding us with its lessons and experiences. Our mistakes and challenges are not chains but stepping stones to growth. By incorporating ancient wisdom into our lives, we honor the past, keep its teachings alive, and ensure it remains relevant in our ever-changing world. Let's preserve and cherish the rich heritage of our elders, creating a legacy of wisdom and understanding for generations to come.

Chapter 6:
Our Partners in the Journey

Understanding my partner's menstrual cycle has brought us closer. It's not just about managing symptoms, but about deepening our empathy and connection. –John

Building Bridges Together—Understanding Each Other's Rhythms

Our moon cycle weaves its gentle rhythm through the fabric of our existence, a delicate thread in the grand tapestry of life. But understanding it goes beyond just biology; it's about empathy, support, and maintaining healthy relationships. As hormones fluctuate throughout our cycle, our needs and emotions change, impacting how we interact with our partners and those around us.

Being comfortable with our changes and communicating throughout our cycle can lead to better intimacy, clearer communication, and a deeper connection. Share with your partner how different phases affect your mood, energy, and desires, fostering mutual understanding and support. Open, transparent, and honest communication, being present for others and being seen ourselves, listening and being heard, and empathy are key to building mutual understanding, deepening connections, and enhancing emotional intimacy. Consider using a shared calendar to track and plan activities according to these phases.

When conflicts arise, mutual understanding makes resolving them easier. Approaching disagreements with empathy and a desire for resolution helps maintain respect and constructive communication. Love thrives on understanding—knowing our partner's strengths, flaws, and being there for them unconditionally. Without it, misunderstandings and frustrations can arise.

As for you, our partners, making your way through the maze of our changing emotional states throughout our cycle requires empathy as your compass, communication as your guiding star, and support as your steadfast anchor. Here are some examples of unspoken languages of love that every woman desires to receive:

- **Let's communicate:** We are willing to talk about our needs and experiences during our cycle. We would like to have a candid conversation about our menstrual cycle to break down taboos, enhance your understanding, and strengthen our relationship, and to discuss how different phases affect our moods, energy, and intimacy.

- **Let's relax:** Let's create a comforting space together by dimming the lights and snuggling under a cozy blanket. This soothing atmosphere helps us overcome discomfort and stress, bringing us closer and fostering relaxation. Consider adding aromatherapy with essential oils known for their calming properties, like lavender or chamomile.

- **Please be patient with us:** Remember that our mood fluctuations are out of our control and we are already doing everything we know to get them under control. Your patience and sensitivity to our changes are invaluable. Your supportive presence means everything to us.

- **We need your support:** We would prefer to share the household chores during this time. Some days we may need you to even take over. It would mean a lot to us if you could offer some comfort, like heating pads or a soothing massage.

- **Craving your love in tracking our needs together:** Let's track the cycle together to understand the ebb and flow of our needs. This helps in planning for intimacy and emotional support accordingly. Let's discuss how to be intimate during different phases, ensuring both of us feel comfortable and connected. (Naarica, 2023).

Communicating Clearly in a Relationship: The Foundation of Understanding

In any relationship, each person has their own way of talking and listening. It's important for us as couples to figure out how to talk to each other in a way that works for us. Good communication takes practice and effort, and it's okay if it's not perfect all the time. We have to remember that our relationship and union is more important than being right. So, it's important to address our needs clearly. Instead of assuming, communicating openly is the key. Being curious and staying curious in relationships help us to find new ways to understand each other and deepen our connection.

Here's the scoop on how to communicate more openly: Make sure to chat freely and clearly, ditching distractions and sharing your thoughts and feelings using "I" statements. When you listen, really tune in with presence and empathy, picking up on both words and body language. Be comfortable to make eye contact and keep it for as long as you are having a conversation; be genuinely interested. And hey, communication is like a muscle—it gets stronger with practice. Encourage each other to speak up, whether it's with words or actions, and be patient as you figure things out together.

To improve our communication skills, we have to start by asking ourselves:

- What's causing tension between us as a couple? Are we really hearing each other out?

- What makes us both feel content and connected?

- What disappoints or hurts us?

- What topics are tough to discuss, and why?

Let's bring these questions into our conversations with our partner, sharing our thoughts openly. Together, we can explore fresh approaches to our communication and discover new paths toward understanding each other better.

- Understanding our communication patterns empowers us within our relationship. We all encounter those sensitive topics that we instinctively shy away from—whether they stir up painful memories or simply make us uncomfortable. In navigating conflicts within a relationship, we can consider these refined strategies:

- Eschew silence as a response; communicate openly instead.

- Fully grasp the context and facts before drawing conclusions.

- Center discussions on realities rather than presumptions.

- Prioritize comprehension and connection over winning the debate.

- Direct conversations toward present solutions and future harmony rather than past grievances.

- Address significant concerns at the outset, allowing lesser issues to find resolution in their wake.

- Voice emotions through personal reflections using phrases like "I feel," avoiding accusatory "You are" statements (*Relationships and Communication*, n.d.).

Emotional intelligence (EQ) plays a crucial role in understanding and navigating our emotional landscapes during our period. How can we enhance our EQ with active listening, recognizing and naming emotions, and practicing empathy? Try these two activities:

- **Active listening exercise:** Partner 1 shares their feelings about their menstrual cycle for five minutes without interruption. Partner 2 listens actively, maintaining eye contact, and then summarizes what they heard, validating partner 1's feelings. Switch roles and repeat.

- **Recognizing and naming emotions:** Both partners list out the emotions they typically feel during the menstrual cycle and discuss how these emotions impact their behavior and interactions. Practice naming these emotions during conversations to build a shared emotional vocabulary.

Understanding Together: Navigating the Realities of Our Period and Fostering Intimacy Through Shared Knowledge

Does it feel like an uphill task, dealing with mood swings and emotional ups and downs throughout your period? Well, you're not alone. Most of us face symptoms like irritability, anxiety, heightened sensitivity, and trouble focusing every month. These changes affect our relationship too, influencing our interactions, communication, and intimacy. That's why it's important to express ourselves and communicate with our partner about how we feel during our period.

Not only does it help them understand what we're going through, but it also opens up a channel for emotional support:

- **Choosing a calm moment for conversation:** It's best to discuss sensitive topics when we're feeling composed and not overly irritable. This setting allows for a more direct and effective conversation without heightened emotions.

- **Cultivating empathy:** In a period conversation, it's important to appreciate our partner's perspective. They may not fully grasp the intensity of what we are experiencing. Demonstrating patience and striving to see things through their eyes deepens mutual understanding and compassion.

- **Educating on emotional and hormonal shifts:** We can enlighten our partner by sharing insights on how our hormones fluctuate wildly throughout the different phases of our cycle, profoundly impacting our emotions, especially a couple of days before our period starts. This would nurture greater compassion and empathy in our experiences.

- **Guiding our partners on how to be there for us:** It's crucial to communicate what kind of support we need when we're dealing with PMS, be it space to breathe or a big, comforting hug.

- **Keeping our partners informed:** It's necessary to update our partner about our feelings as we notice the first signs of PMS. A quick heads-up can prepare them on the best ways to support us during these times.

Instead of creating distance between us, periods can be a time to deepen our bond. By embracing the strategies listed below, we can use our cycle to deepen and strengthen our relationship

- **Educational involvement:** Both partners can learn more about the menstrual cycle together. This shared knowledge can help in planning and responding to needs more effectively, reducing misunderstandings and increasing support. Attend workshops or read books on the topic together to enhance your collective understanding.

- **Shared self-care:** Practicing self-care routines together (especially during periods), such as relaxing with a warm bath, using heating pads, or practicing yoga, not only provides physical comfort but also enhances emotional bonding and mutual care.

- **Volunteering together on menstrual-cycle-related projects:** By working side by side to support causes like period hygiene, we can improve our shared sense of purpose and compassion. This joint effort can lead to richer conversations, mutual respect, and a greater appreciation for each other.

- **Emotional check-ins:** Schedule regular emotional check-ins to discuss how each partner is feeling and what support they need. This can be particularly helpful during the more emotionally intense phases of the cycle.

- **Expressing appreciation:** Regularly acknowledge and appreciate each other's support and understanding during different phases of the cycle.

- **Stress management:** If mood swings during different phases of the cycle are creating stress, work together with to identify the sources and find solutions. Be open to seeking help if needed, and support each other through the challenges.

Some of the activities that couples can do together to better understand the period and its impact include:

- Reading a book on the subject and sharing insights with each other during a dedicated discussion time.

- Watching educational videos or a documentary about menstrual health and discussing it afterward.

- Attending a workshop on menstrual health and relationship dynamics together.

Supporting Each Other

Offering genuine emotional support means extending kindness and respect to those who need it. For all our partners looking to support us during our periods, the key is to be present and attentive. Presence is everything in a relationship. Consider keeping a journal to note patterns and understand each other's responses better over time. It's important to tune into our needs and offer care and understanding.

Emotional Support Techniques

- **Predict and prepare:** Understanding our cycle is the key. Ourselves and our partners could utilize a period-tracking app with sharing options to stay aware and be prepared to offer help when needed.

- **Indulging our cravings:** Cravings are a very common part of our monthly experience. Stock up on comforting treats like our favourite chocolate, tea, or whatever we prefer.

A little indulgence can go a long way and will be greatly appreciated.

• **Please be present and attentive:** Especially when talking to others who haven't experienced a period, it's important to handle these conversations with maturity. Avoid showing insensitivity in various ways and making assumptions. Just listen—we might not want to chat, but if we do, be there without judging.

• **Respect our space:** Before assuming we want to be alone, kindly check in with us first in a nonjudgmental way. If we do prefer solitude, staying in touch through texts to show you care can mean a lot..

• **Easing the hurt together:** Keep a water bottle nearby so we can stay hydrated and refill it when it's low. Encourage light yoga, especially staying in child's pose, with wide legs and a pillow underneath us to hug, or taking a walk outside to ease PMS and cramps, but don't force it if we're not feeling up to it.

• **Distract and relax:** Keep us entertained with our favorite shows to score some brownie points and bond together. Search the list of uplifting Period Positive Films.

• **TLC time—spoil us right:** Treat us like royalty with massages, candlelit baths, and homemade dinners. Help out with chores and errands to ease our stress and let us relax. Even if we're not in much pain, we will appreciate the effort and feel loved.

• **Hang in there:** This time can be super emotional, hitting some of us harder than others. Remember, everyone handles periods differently, so welcome our differences. And never, ever call us "crazy"—it will only make things worse :). Stay present. Let's meditate together, it will be good for both of us. Things will settle down, and our relationship will stay strong (*8 Ways You Can Support Your Partner,* n.d.).

Overcoming Challenges Together

Period taboos because of misconceptions are still a thing in many cultures, leading to women and girls being excluded from various roles. These false beliefs fuel stigma and shame, with some believing periods to be impure or unclean. This leads to exclusion from basic facilities, hindering social participation.

Change is tough for everyone, and it's even harder when it comes to menstrual health stuff. If we can't talk openly about periods in schools or in the workplace, it's tough to make any progress. When men get called to a period training session, they often ask why they're there. But this resistance puts girls at risk because they miss out on the support and info they need.

- **Create awareness in both boys and girls:** Teach them about puberty, pain relief, and hygiene. Help boys understand the menstrual cycle so they can support and connect girls with the right help when needed.

- **Bust myths and taboos:** Talking about periods, cultures, and beliefs can help both boys and girls see that menstruation is totally normal.

- **Understanding menstrual disorders:** Learning about issues like endometriosis or heavy flows helps men understand why periods can be tough. It also makes them more likely to support their partners and daughters by providing what they need for better care and understanding their health better.

• **Period problems and solutions:** Girls and women often get sidelined during their periods, sometimes even getting banished from basic activities like cooking or bathing. This taboo significantly undermines self-esteem. But talking about periods is key. Let's break the pattern and create a new imprint. From rookies to period pros, everyone benefits from keeping the convo going. Discussion topics for couples include the importance of menstrual health education for both partners, and how cultural taboos and misconceptions about menstruation can be challenged and changed within the relationship and the wider community.

• **Talk to the doctor:** Got period worries? Chat with a doc. There might be ways to make our monthly visitor a bit more bearable.

• **Dealing with PMS:** Straight couples can hit some bumps during PMS week. Women organically feel more sensitive and may even tend to create relationship problems just because of hormonal fluctuations, which can lead to conflicts. So, when we're dealing with PMS, take it seriously, but take us lightly (Brown, 2021).

Communication is key in tackling challenges together. Being open and supportive can really help ease the stress. That's the real support we need.

Empowering Our Partners

Empowerment means lifting each other up instead of holding each other down. It's like being each other's cheerleaders! Instead of fighting for power through manipulation and control, we support and encourage our partner. When both partners empower each other, the relationship is stronger and happier.

Heads-up for our partners: To empower us, you can do small things like giving us hugs and kisses, or holding hands. These simple gestures make us feel loved and connected. Sending messages of love and support throughout the day also helps us to stay connected, especially during tough times. It's all about showing love and kindness to make each other feel great!

Empowering us also means being there for us when we're going through a tough time. Sometimes, all we need is someone to listen and understand without judging or giving advice. It's like putting yourself in our shoes and trying to see things from our perspective, even if it's different from yours. We can agree to disagree and hold space for our differences. Even if we don't totally get each other's opinions, ideas, or dreams, it is powerful for us to make the effort to understand each other and connect on a deeper level.

And don't forget, part of empowerment is cheering us on to be the best we can be! Being in a committed relationship means mutual respect and equality, effective communication, growth and support, shared responsibilities, emotional intimacy, commitment to working through challenges, and continuous effort. It starts with both partners being willing to invest in and nurture the relationship, recognizing that love and connection require ongoing dedication and understanding.

In almost all relationships, one partner can see the other's strengths and weaknesses better than they can see it themselves. This is the magic of being in a relationship—letting our partner show us how awesome we are and encourage us to go for it! Being supportive means lifting us up when we're feeling low, helping out with stuff when we're chasing our dreams, and celebrating our successes. The magic really happens when both partners support each other to the point that both feel heard, seen, accepted, and welcomed. Things may take time, but good things take time :). Throughout our lives together, we will have many opportunities to grow, helping each other chase our dreams—both those we share and those we have on our own.

Role of Advocacy

Period advocacy groups have played a pivotal role in creating awareness about menstrual health, which has a deep impact on interpersonal relationships, especially with partners. By educating the public and breaking down the stigma associated with menstruation, these groups contribute toward an environment of openness and understanding. This awareness has a direct influence on the strength of bonds between partners in several key ways:

- **Shared responsibilities:** Awareness campaigns often emphasize the importance of shared responsibilities in maintaining period hygiene. Partners who are educated about menstrual health are more likely to contribute to tasks such as purchasing period products or ensuring a clean and comfortable environment. This collaborative approach can strengthen the partnership by promoting equality and mutual respect.

- **Reducing misconceptions and taboos:** Period advocacy breaks down long-standing misconceptions and taboos surrounding menstruation. When partners are freed from these stigmas, they can approach the topic with a more positive and supportive attitude. This shift in perspective can reduce tension and foster a more harmonious relationship.

By promoting education and open dialogue about menstrual health, these groups help partners build stronger, more empathetic, and more supportive bonds. The emphasis on period hygiene as part of these advocacy efforts ensures that partners are not only better informed but also more engaged in maintaining a healthy and respectful relationship dynamic.

Celebrating Togetherness

Here are some ways to celebrate togetherness in a way that is centered around the female partner's menstrual cycle:

- **Regular communication:** Keeping communication channels open during the menstrual cycle helps partners bond and feel appreciated. Discussing feelings, symptoms, and needs shows care and helps both partners stay aligned and connected.

- **Asking for feedback:** Asking for ideas on how to better support each other during this time demonstrates respect, openness, and dedication. Inviting insights on managing menstrual symptoms and emotional needs shows that you value your partner's perspective and are committed to enhancing the relationship.

- **Intimate gestures:** Small, thoughtful actions can make a big difference. For example, preparing a cozy environment with her favorite snacks and a heating pad and binge-watching a beloved show together can provide comfort and show that you're thinking of her.

- **Paying compliments:** Genuine compliments can boost your partner's mood and self-esteem, especially during her period. Saying things like, "You always make our home so cozy and inviting" can make her feel cherished and appreciated.

- **Honoring feelings:** Actively listening to your partner when she shares her excitement or frustration during the ebb and flow of emotions is essential. Take her feelings seriously and offer empathy and support rather than brushing them off.

- **Living in the present:** Instead of stressing over future scenarios, focus on the present. What can you do together right now to strengthen your relationship? Engaging in activities that bring joy and relaxation can help both partners feel more connected. For example, set up a cozy corner with blankets, pillows, and aromatic candles or incense and play soothing music to create a calming atmosphere in which you can both relax.

- **Daily love and appreciation:** Strengthen your bond by showing love and appreciation every day, not just during periods or right before a period when she is feeling down. Ensure that both partners feel acknowledged, listened to, and cherished year-round. Simple daily acts of kindness and recognition go a long way in maintaining a healthy and loving relationship.

By embracing these practices and celebrating the menstrual cycle together, partners can build a deeper connection, enhance their understanding of each other, and nurture a more supportive and loving relationship.

Conclusion: Stronger Together

Our social connections play a big role in our well-being, affecting both our happiness and our health. Loneliness and isolation can lead to poor mental and physical health, while good-quality relationships can boost our mood and even extend our lives. Mood swings during our periods can be challenging, but understanding and communication help maintain the strength of the bond between partners. We have to make an effort to openly talk to our partners, explaining how our being irritable and moody is the result of the change in our hormone levels. They care about us and will support us through tough times with understanding, without judgment or blame.

To keep our relationships strong and healthy, we should view challenges as opportunities to grow, avoid blaming each other, and learn from past mistakes. Respecting each other's feelings by accepting and embracing all emotions, even the difficult ones like anger or jealousy, is essential.

By following these tips, we can nurture deeper intimacy and avoid common pitfalls like blame and shame that can harm relationships.

Chapter 7:
Wellness Practices

Aligning Everyday Wellness With Our Cycle

Well-being involves feeling good, functioning well, and handling life's stresses. It includes life satisfaction, purpose, and control. Factors like exercise, diet, relationships, career, self-care, spirituality, finances, and the living environment all contribute to overall well-being.

Wellness means practicing healthy habits daily for better physical and mental health. Simple, healthy choices can reduce stress, enhance social interactions, and improve overall wellness.

Hormonal changes during the menstrual cycle affect sleep, sex drive, energy, and mood, impacting well-being. "Cycle syncing" helps us adjust to these natural changes by adapting lifestyle habits aligned to the four phases of the menstrual cycle, including changes to our workout routines, diet, and sex life.

To start cycle syncing, using a period-tracking app is recommended. Here are some tips:

- **Create your own path:** Understand the common signs and symptoms of each phase, but remember your experience is unique.

- **Track symptoms:** Record your symptoms in an app or a journal for a few months to spot patterns and adjust your habits accordingly.

- **Listen to your body:** Tune into your emotional, physical, and mental needs and trust your intuition.

Wellness Practices for Each Phase

Incorporating yoga and mindful eating into my routine has transformed my menstrual experience. I feel more balanced, both physically and emotionally. –Emily

Spring—Maiden or Virgin Phase Wellness

Breath Work for Renewal

Breath work techniques can invigorate and energize the body and mind, preparing us for a new cycle. "Breath of fire" is a breathing technique with passive inhalations and forceful, rapid exhalations that involve contracting the abdominal muscles. This method revitalizes us by enhancing brain function. The inhalation and exhalation are equal in length, with no pause in between. The focus is on the breathing pattern rather than the speed, so beginners should start slowly and increase the pace gradually. Performed seated, breath of fire sessions can last from 30 seconds to 10 minutes, depending on your experience and preference.

In addition to breath of fire, you can try "box breathing," which involves inhaling for four counts, holding for four counts, exhaling for four counts, and holding for four counts. This is ideal for calming the mind and body.

If it's been a while since you practiced breath work, "lion's breath" would be the best technique for you: Inhale deeply, then exhale forcefully with a roaring sound to release tension.

Meditation for Clarity and Vision

Manifestation meditation is ideal during the Maiden phase of our cycle. This practice involves concentrating intently on something through our third eye, located between our eyebrows, to stay present and quiet our mind. A good focus point is our breath, as it's a common entry into meditation.

Setting our intentions is essential for our meditation practice. Intentions are our true nodes, reminding us where we are heading when we feel confused or lost. They are essential in our human journey, helping us stay on track.

Instructions

1. **Get comfortable and sit upright:** If you're on a chair, sit on the edge with your feet on the floor. If you're on the ground, use a cushion or block to relax your thighs and keep your spine straight.
2. **Relax your body:** Drop your shoulders and breathe from your belly. The key is to keep your body upright, let your head just follow your spine, and be very comfortable, just sitting. Here, we just deepen our inhalations, keeping a soft belly, and exhale completely each time.
3. **Focus on your intention:** See your intention through the third eye. Start building an image, paying attention to its sound, smell, sight, and any other details you notice. Don't think about it—just experience it and stay present. Observe your breath, noticing the sensations of each inhale and exhale.
4. **Quiet your inner voice:** When your mind starts wandering, gently bring your attention back to the breath and the intention. You don't have a goal; it's all about the experience.
5. **Don't stress about perfection:** When you notice your mind drifting, instead of criticizing yourself, just stay with the breath. This will help you return to the present moment.

Yoga Posture for Activation

During the follicular phase, it's best to choose a yoga pose that boosts energy flow, like Sun Salutation. This dynamic sequence not only builds muscle but also enhances flexibility and gets our blood flowing. We start standing and then move through poses that stretch, strengthen, and energize us.

Instructions

1. **Start in Mountain Pose:** Stand tall with your feet grounded and arms relaxed by your sides.
2. **Reach up:** Inhale deeply and sweep your arms overhead, palms facing each other. Lift your chest toward the sky.
3. **Fold forward:** Exhale slowly, bending at your hips to fold forward. Keep your spine straight and your hands on the floor or close to your feet.
4. **Halfway lift:** Inhale again, lifting your torso to a flat back position. Reach forward with your head and keep your chest parallel to the ground.
5. **Plank pose:** Exhale as you step or jump back to a plank position. Keep your body straight, with your wrists under your shoulders and your core engaged (Ezrin, 2022).

Nourishment and Nutrition

To promote better estrogen metabolism in this phase, we should opt for cabbage, kale, broccoli, and leafy greens. To boost iron, we can use organic fish or a Lucky Iron Fish, which is a simple cooking tool designed to add a significant portion of our daily required iron intake when added to any boiling liquids for 10 minutes. To enhance iron absorption, citrus fruits work miracles. It is advisable to keep our meals light and fresh, adding probiotic-rich foods like fermented veggies (e.g., sauerkraut). Our body will certainly thank us!

Example Meal Ideas

- **Breakfast:** Smoothie with kale, pineapple, mango, flaxseeds, cayenne, and coconut water

- **Lunch:** Buckwheat salad with mixed greens, cherry tomatoes, cucumber, avocado, and a light vinaigrette

- **Snack:** Veggie sticks (carrots, celery, cucumber) with hummus

- **Dinner:** Stir-fried tempeh with leafy greens, asparagus, bell peppers, snap peas, carrots, garlic, ginger, and tamari

Essential Oils for the Maiden

During the follicular phase, we should raise our inner warrior with yang oils to help us stay active and accomplish tasks:

- **Cardamom:** Enhances focus and restores energy.

- **Basil:** Clears the mind and aids decision-making; it also helps reduce fatigue and supports adrenal function.

- **Ginger:** Fuels determination and creativity.

- **Peppermint and rosemary:** Improve intellect and emotional resilience.

- **Melissa (lemon balm):** Helps uplift mood, reduces anxiety, and supports cognitive function.

Summer—Mother Phase Wellness

Breath Work for Connection

During the ovulatory phase, we should try a breathing exercise that brings warmth and openness, like the 4-7-8 breath technique. This technique can effectively calm the mind and prepare the body for nurturing activities. It's simple: Count as you breathe in and out. Breathe in for a count of four, hold your breath for seven counts, then release it over eight counts. This helps calm our mind and fully empty our lungs. Couples can practice the 4-7-8 breath together by sitting and facing each other, holding hands or maintaining eye contact; this leads to the two partners synchronizing breaths for increased connection and calmness.

Meditation for Empathy and Love

In the summer phase, Buddha's *metta bhavana* meditation is perfect. It cultivates loving-kindness and goodwill toward ourselves, loved ones, acquaintances, difficult individuals, and, ultimately, all beings.

Instructions

1. Posture is everything. The key is to sit as straight as possible and find your comfort.
2. Imagine someone you deeply love sitting across from you, connected heart to heart by a glowing white light. Let the warmth and affection you feel for them fill your body.
3. Now, focus on the words "Let me be well, in peace and be happy," feeling the loving-kindness within you.
4. Send these feelings to your friend, saying, "I wish you are happy, in peace, and keeping well."

5. As you breathe naturally, feel the connection between the two of you as you repeat the phrases silently.
6. Imagine the white light expanding into a circle around you, spreading warmth and peace to all beings, big and small, across the universe.
7. Continue silently repeating the phrases, feeling the warmth and expansion within you.
8. Take a moment to notice your feelings and sensations without judgment, then slowly open your eyes (Nash, 2024).

Yoga Posture for Strength

During the Mother phase, a great pose for stability and strength is Warrior II (Virabhadrasana II). This pose helps improve stamina, increase flexibility in the body and the mind, enhance balance, and improve mental focus.

Instructions

1. Stand at the top of your mat.
2. Step your left foot back about 4 feet, turning it out to a 90-degree angle. Keep your right foot facing forward.
3. Ensure your right heel aligns with the arch of your left foot.
4. Bend your right knee over your right ankle, making sure your thigh is parallel to the floor. Avoid letting your knee extend beyond your ankle.
5. Press firmly into both feet and engage your leg muscles.
6. Lift your torso upright, ensuring your hips are square to the side.
7. Raise your arms to your sides, parallel to the floor, palms facing down. Reach actively from fingertip to fingertip.
8. Turn your head to gaze over your right hand, keeping your

shoulders relaxed and your gaze steady.

9. Hold this position for 30 seconds to 1 minute, breathing deeply and maintaining your alignment and engagement. Practice using affirmations such as "I am," "I can," and "I will" to increase your mental and emotional resilience.
10. Straighten your right leg and lower your arms.
11. Repeat the pose on the other side by turning your left foot out and bending your left knee.

Nourishing Foods and Herbs

During ovulation, we should focus on nutrient-rich foods to support fertility, such as:

- Folate-rich foods like leafy greens, citrus fruits, and beans for better cell division.

- Healthy fats to boost hormone production—an avocado a day makes life just better!

- Omega-3-rich foods like salmon, chia seeds, and flaxseeds are also beneficial.

Our high estrogen levels during ovulation can reduce our appetite and increase our energy levels, so we should:

- Prioritize proteins, fats, and fiber for sustained energy and hormone balance.

- Choose fiber-packed veggies like asparagus, Brussels sprouts, and spinach.

- Eat antioxidant-rich fruits like raspberries, strawberries, coconut, and guava for liver detoxification.

- Opt for lighter carbs like quinoa and amaranth.

- Add nuts and seeds like sunflower seeds, almonds, and sesame seeds for extra nutrients.

Example Meal Ideas

- **Breakfast:** Smoothie with spinach, chia seeds, berries, and almond milk

- **Lunch:** Grilled wild-caught salmon with black quinoa and steamed vegetables

- **Snack:** Unsweetened and unflavoured soya yogurt with raw honey and organic activated nuts

- **Dinner:** Stir-fried tofu with broccoli, carrots, and wild rice

Essential Oils for the Mother Phase

During ovulation, floral and earthy oils make for a delightful experience. Examples include:

- **Cypress:** Improves circulation and can help reduce any bloating or water retention.

- **Black pepper:** Stimulates circulation and provides an energizing effect.

- **Neroli:** Supports hormonal balance, reduces stress, and enhances mood.

Autumn—Witch Phase Wellness

Breath Work for Grounding

In the autumn phase, we crave a breath work technique that will steady our changing emotions, like alternate nostril breathing. This breathing technique balances the nervous system and stabilizes our emotions. We begin by closing our right nostril with our right thumb, then we breathe in through our left nostril and hold. We then switch, closing our left nostril with our right index finger as we exhale through our right nostril. Then we pause before repeating the sequence. As we breathe in through our left nostril, let's visualize drawing in light and grounding energy. As we exhale through our right nostril, visualize releasing tension and stress. This method helps bring balance to both our mind and our body.

Meditation for Self-Reflection

During the luteal phase, we should try a meditation method that promotes self-reflection and emotional understanding, like mindfulness meditation. This is a practice where we focus on the present moment without judgment. Instead of trying to alter our emotions, we learn to observe them as they are and accept them without resistance.

Instructions

1. Get comfortable wherever you're sitting—whether it's a chair, cushion, or bench. Make sure you're stable, not perched or slouching.
2. Cross your legs comfortably if you're on a cushion, or let your feet touch the floor if you're in a chair or on a bench.

3. Untuck your pelvis, soften your belly, and elongate your spine, with your head and shoulders resting comfortably.
4. Position your upper arms parallel to your body and let your hands rest on your legs. Find the right balance—not too far forward, not too far back.
5. Lower your chin slightly and let your gaze fall gently downward.
6. Relax for a moment and bring your focus to your breath or the sensations in your body.
7. Feel your breath, and observe how it goes in and out. Pay attention to how it feels in your nose, mouth, belly, and chest.
8. Before making any movements, pause and consider them intentionally, slowing down completely. Shift your position with awareness.
9. Our minds are made to wander, so welcome it. You can notice your thoughts without becoming entangled in them.
10. When you're ready, lift your gaze and take a moment to notice your surroundings, how your body feels, and your thoughts (Mindful Staff, 2023).

Yoga Posture for Balance

During the autumn phase, we seek yoga poses that help us find both physical and emotional balance—like Vrksasana, also known as Tree Pose. It improves balance, strength, and stability in our legs as well as concentration and awareness as we stabilize ourselves.

Instructions

1. Start in a standing or mountain pose, keeping your shoulders relaxed, back straight, and feet together.
2. Focus on a spot in front of you, breathing deeply and staying

still.

3. Exhale and raise your right leg, placing the foot on the inside of your left thigh. Keep your standing leg straight and your core engaged.
4. Inhale and raise your arms overhead, palms together in a prayer position.
5. Hold the pose for three to five breaths, maintaining balance and awareness.
6. Exhale and lower your arms, returning to standing.
7. Repeat with your left leg, placing the foot on the inside of your right thigh.
8. Hold the pose for three to five breaths, focusing on balance and breathing (Lynette, n.d.).

Nourishing Practices

During our autumn phase, we should eat foods rich in beta-carotene like leafy greens, carrots, and sweet potatoes to support hormone regulation and cell growth. Pineapple, with its bromelain content, can also boost fertility by aiding egg implantation.

To avoid emotional ups and downs from skipping meals, it is better to eat regularly (every three to four hours).

Progesterone levels during this phase can cause constipation and bloating. These symptoms are combated with foods high in B vitamins, calcium, magnesium complex, and fiber, like psyllium husk, and roasted starchy vegetables such as sweet potatoes and squash.

It is advisable to choose buckwheat and millet as grains and include protein sources like bone broth and liver.

For hormonal balance, sipping peppermint tea or adding marine algae like spirulina to our smoothies is a good option.

- **Breakfast:** Gluten-free oatmeal with flaxseed, banana, and sugar-free almond butter

- **Lunch:** Lentil soup with a side of mixed greens

- **Snack:** Apple slices with cinnamon, tajin, or hummus with cayenne

- **Dinner:** Baked sweet potato with black beans, avocado, and a sprinkle of lime juice with Celtic sea salt

Essential Oils for the Witch

During the luteal phase, essential oils like geranium, bergamot, lavender, and palmarosa can help manage PMS by releasing pent-up emotions and clearing the mind:

- **Vetiver:** Grounds emotions, reduces stress, and promotes restful sleep.
- **Bergamot:** Prevents fatigue and depression by dispersing stagnant energy.
- **Lavender:** Soothes frustration and irritability, promoting relaxation.
- **Marjoram:** Eases muscle tension and pain and helps with relaxation.
- **Patchouli:** Promotes relaxation, reduces stress, and balances mood.

Winter—Wise Woman Phase Wellness

Breath Work for Release

During the wise woman phase, it's beneficial to practice deep, releasing breath work to help transition from the old cycle. One effective technique is deep abdominal breathing, which helps us to release physical and emotional tension, promoting relaxation. With this method, we take a long, deep breath, visualizing it filling our entire body. As we inhale, we allow our belly and chest to expand. Upon exhaling, we feel our chest relax and our navel draw back toward our spine. This deep breathing signals our body to relax and let go. While practicing deep abdominal breathing, visualize a peaceful place where you feel safe and relaxed. Imagine yourself there, absorbing the zen environment with each breath.

Meditation for Insight

In the wise woman phase, insight meditation, also known as Vipassana, helps in understanding the nature of our experiences for profound wisdom. The three stages of insight in meditation involve recognizing our mental and physical processes, understanding their impermanent nature, and realizing nonattachment to these processes.

Instructions

1. Set aside 10–15 minutes for practice, whenever you need when you are bleeding.
2. Choose a quiet area with minimal distractions, like an empty room or a secluded spot outside.
3. Ideally, sit comfortably on the ground in a cross-legged position. However, if needed, depending on how your period

is treating you, you can lie down. Whether sitting or lying down, keep your back straight, relax your body, and soften your hips and belly.

4. Close your eyes and breathe naturally. Focus on your breath and any sensations you feel.

5. Observe each inhale and exhale, including your thoughts and feelings, without judgment.

6. If you get distracted, acknowledge it and return to your breath.

7. Start with 5–10 minutes and gradually increase to 15 minutes or more as you become accustomed to the practice (Huxter, n.d.).

Yoga Posture for Rest

Winter is all about cozying up and taking it easy. When it comes to yoga, there's a perfect match for that vibe: restorative yoga. Since the focus is on relaxation and not breaking a sweat, we can let go of tension in our muscles without any discomfort creeping in.

Child's pose is very restorative and great for relieving stress and fatigue. It gently stretches our spine, hips, glutes, hamstrings, and shoulder muscles.

Instructions for Child's Pose

1. Start by kneeling on the floor with your knees apart and your toes touching the ground. Sit back on your heels.

2. If you need extra support, you can slide a cushion or folded blanket between your thighs and calves.

3. Take a deep breath, then exhale and lean forward, lowering your torso between your thighs until your forehead touches the floor.

4. Stretch your arms out in front of you, or if that's too much, you can let them relax by your sides with your palms facing up.

5. For even more comfort, you can rest your head and arms on a cushion or folded blanket.

6. Stay in this cozy pose for a minimum of 5 minutes, breathing deeply and relaxing. If you have cramps, you can get into this posture, take a pillow or cushion to hug, and try to sleep this way.

7. When you're ready to come out of child's pose, slowly lift your torso back up until you're in a seated position (Lindberg, 2020).

Additional Restorative Poses for the Winter

- **Supported bridge pose:** Lie on your back with a bolster or pillow under your lower back.

- **Reclined butterfly pose:** Lie on your back with the soles of your feet together and knees apart, supported by pillows or blocks.

Nourishing Foods and Herbs

During our period, we should focus on replenishing nutrients and easing discomfort. Iron-rich foods like spinach and lentils combat fatigue, while protein-rich foods like fish and beans ease cramps and prevent anemia for heavy bleeders. Warm foods to warm our belly, such as homemade soups, would be perfect.

Opting for comforting cooking methods and ingredients like warm soups, bone broth, stir-fries, and sea vegetables is recommended. Antioxidant-rich smoothies with dark berries, kale, and flaxseed are beneficial for hormone balance and inflammation reduction, as is dark chocolate.

Example Meal Ideas

- **Breakfast:** Iron-fortified organic gluten-free oats with blueberries and a splash of almond milk

- **Lunch:** Lentil and spinach stew with whole-grain bread

- **Snack:** Trail mix with organic sugar-free dark chocolate, nuts, and dried fruit

- **Dinner:** Baked wild-caught salmon with roasted sweet potatoes and steamed broccoli

Essential Oils for the Wise Woman

During menstruation, we should use oils like lavender, rose, geranium, bergamot, sandalwood, frankincense, clary sage, and thyme for introspection and relaxation:

- **Frankincense:** Offers anti-inflammatory properties, helps with pain relief, supports emotional grounding, promotes tranquility, and eases cramps.

- **Lavender, rose, and bergamot:** Help with relaxation and pain relief, ease emotional tension, and promote feelings of comfort and love..

- **Blue tansy:** Known for its anti-inflammatory properties, blue tansy helps reduce pain and promotes emotional well-being.

- **Thyme:** Another effective pain reliever.

Personalized Wellness Practices for Each Phase

Personalized wellness practices can significantly improve our experience of each phase of our menstrual cycle. These simple personalized wellness plans should include specific activities, foods, and self-care practices tailored to the unique needs of each phase:

Spring (Maiden/Virgin Phase)

- **Activities:** Gentle cardio, creative projects, social engagements
- **Foods:** Fresh salads, citrus fruits, lean proteins
- **Self-care:** Journaling, vision boarding, skincare rituals

Summer (Mother Phase)

- **Activities:** High-energy workouts, community events, volunteering
- **Foods:** Nutrient-dense meals, healthy fats, protein-rich snacks
- **Self-care:** Aromatherapy, spa days, outdoor activities

Autumn (Witch Phase)

- **Activities:** Restorative yoga, nature walks, introspective activities
- **Foods:** Warm, comforting meals, complex carbs, herbal teas
- **Self-care:** Meditation, essential oil baths, reading

Winter (Wise Woman Phase):

- **Activities:** Restorative practices, minimal physical exertion, quiet time
- **Foods:** Iron-rich foods, warming soups, dark chocolate
- **Self-care:** Hot baths, deep breathing exercises, cozy blankets

Conclusion: Integrating Practices Into Daily Life

Menstrual cycle syncing, or hormonal syncing, is a self-care practice where we as women align lifestyle elements like diet and exercise with our menstrual cycle to maximize wellness. The concept involves adjusting our daily routines to match the natural hormonal changes during the menstrual cycle's four phases. This helps address energy levels, physical changes, and mood fluctuations.

Syncing involves tuning into our body to understand what foods and activities make us feel our best. Benefits may include improved mood, hormone balance, energy, and productivity, as well as relief from PMS symptoms.

Once we understand our cycle's length and symptoms, we can tailor our lifestyle choices accordingly. We should try syncing our workouts, which involves adjusting our exercise routines based on the hormonal changes in each phase of the menstrual cycle. Syncing can also extend to our dietary choices, prioritizing certain foods and increasing hydration to ease menstrual symptoms and provide the body with optimal fuel. We can start by tracking our cycle with an app like Flo or Clue. We can then experiment with adjusting our diet, exercise, and self-care practices based on the phases of our cycle, and can also join online communities or workshops focused on cycle syncing to share experiences and gain additional insights.

We must give cycle syncing a try to reap its benefits; it doesn't cost much, but it holds great promise.

Chapter 8:
Celebrating Every Phase Like a Movement

Embracing Our Inner Dance

We're totally in sync with nature, and our bodies have their own rhythms. For those of us with wombs, this rhythm comes with a special mix of hormones that makes us feel different and give us unique abilities.

Just like any natural cycle, our menstrual cycle has its ups and downs. If we learn to go with the flow instead of fighting it, we can really tap into its power. By tuning into our cycle and recognizing the four female archetypes, we can celebrate the divine feminine both inside and out. This helps us notice and enjoy the subtle shifts in our femininity, each one bringing its own special gifts.

Understanding these four female archetypes starts with getting to know our menstrual cycle. Our mood swings, energy changes, and shifting desires aren't random or irrational—they're part of a natural, powerful rhythm. But our cycle isn't just a biological process; it's a journey that unlocks different archetypal aspects of ourselves. Each phase gifts us with unique abilities and taps into shared psychological traits we all possess:

- **Maiden phase superpowers:** curiosity and fun
- **Mother phase superpowers:** nurturing and relishing
- **Witch phase superpowers:** artistry and gut feeling
- **Wise Woman phase superpowers:** insight and surrender

Just as each person is unique, each archetype has its own set of needs and gifts. It's like we're conducting a complex symphony within ourselves, where understanding the notes can deeply enhance our self-care. It's not about avoiding bad days altogether, but about their frequency and finding more productive, peaceful days in between. We have to understand that our bodies are not out there troubling us; they are just following a natural rhythm. If we learn to accept, welcome, and follow that rhythm, we will be supporting our body. The key is that by embracing these phases, we can empower ourselves to ride the wave of our life and cycle with care.

A word of caution for all women: It's not about perfection; it's about progress and figuring out what works best for us. We are the journey.

In this chapter, we'll explore practical tips for managing our activities during the four phases of our cycle. By arming ourselves with knowledge and taking a holistic approach, we can move through our menstrual cycle with more ease and embrace our natural flow.

Spring—Celebrating New Beginnings

The Maiden's Awakening

The Maiden is linked to the waxing moon and follicular phase (like springtime). She's youthful, full of hope and energy, and a carefree spirit. She's all about being independent, strong, and sure of herself.

People also call her the Virgin because she's pure in mind. She's a woman who's free, sexually independent, and not controlled by anyone. The Maiden remains resolute, firmly grounded in her innate strength. She naturally draws toward herself desired elements—individuals, opportunities, and endeavors. A woman who embodies the Maiden archetype radiates with brilliance, establishing a profound connection with the cosmos and sensing its guidance.

As spring arrives, it brings with it a surge of renewal, energy, and vitality. The Maiden feels a rush of optimism, sparking heightened creativity and a desire for increased social connection. Emotions soar, lifting mood and enhancing overall well-being.

Let's honor and celebrate this time of growth and preparation as we journey through our menstrual cycle with renewed vitality and joy. This phase beckons us to embrace our newfound strength and enthusiasm by participating in rituals that resonate with the heightened vigor of our bodies.

Activities and Celebrations

During the Maiden phase, our hormones line up with what society typically expects from us. We're sharp, able to learn and get things done, predictable, and focused on the outside world. It's like our brains are super-ready to soak up new knowledge and tackle challenges:

- **Let's set up goals:** This phase is all about clarity and focus, so whether it's big dreams or small steps, this is our time to map out our plans and start moving toward them.

- **Lets connect with nature:** Let's take leisurely park strolls, explore trails, or simply chill surrounded by greenery to ground ourselves, breathe in fresh air, and marvel at nature's wonders.

- **Let's be more active:** Our body is bursting with energy, making this phase ideal for invigorating physical activities. Let's embrace this vitality with light cardio exercises like brisk walking, jogging, or dancing to refresh both body and mind.

- **Lets activate our social calendar:** Plan outings, gatherings, or fun activities with friends and family. Let's seek joy and fulfillment through social connections and group activities.

- **Unleashing our creativity:** Let's engage in activities like painting, crafting, or writing to harness our heightened creativity. This is a great time for innovative ideas and fresh perspectives.

- **Let's be grateful:** Reflecting on what we appreciate in our life increases our overall contentment.

- **Learning something new:** Let's engage in activities that stimulate our mind and creativity, such as starting a new hobby, taking a class, or reading an inspiring book.

- **Organizing spaces:** Let's use our surge of energy to declutter and organize our home or workspace, creating a fresh and inviting environment.

Rituals Honoring the Maiden

- Buying flowers for ourselves.

- Starting each day with a short meditation.

- Moving our bodies again.

- Journaling about this cycle's commitments with love and intention.

- Getting into planning mode and defining concrete actions to make our intentions happen.

- Putting on some music and allowing ourselves to move and dance freely.

- Ending our super-active day with an evening routine of a short meditation and a gratitude practice.

• Starting a journal to capture our thoughts, dreams, and plans for the future, using it as a space for reflection and goal setting.

• Taking part in outdoor activities to spend time in nature, whether it's a hike, a picnic, or simply sitting in a park to reconnect with the earth and our inner self.

Summer—Embracing Full Bloom

The Mother's Embrace

The Mother archetype aligns with the full moon and ovulatory phase, symbolizing creativity, nurturing, and attentiveness.

Often reduced to childbearing and rearing, the Mother archetype embodies much more. She nurtures without controlling, offering support for growth and allowing freedom for independence. True creation involves co-creating with the divine, cultivating something that can thrive independently.

Deeply connected to the earth and all life forms, she believes that nurturing ourselves also nourishes Mother Earth. Caring for ourselves helps honor and heal the planet, as everything is interconnected.

Many of us focus our nurturing energy outward—toward children, family, and community—neglecting our own needs. However, self-care is crucial; we can't light the way with an empty lantern. Taking care of ourselves isn't a luxury but a fundamental necessity.

In the summer phase, we naturally lean toward taking care of others, wanting everyone to feel good and content. We are at the peak of our cycle and feel strong, confident, and super social. It's a prime time to tap into our natural charisma and focus our energy on activities that make us feel alive and vibrant.

Activities and Celebrations

- **Celebrating our sensuality:** This is a great time to embrace our femininity and express ourselves. Let's try rituals that celebrate our body and its desires and dress up in clothes that make us feel amazing.

- **Embracing our community connection:** It's also the perfect time to reach out to our community to share our stories and dreams. Let's host a get-together with friends, throw a dinner party, or organize a fun activity together.

- **Strengthening personal connections:** Let's start heart-to-heart chats, enjoy quality moments with loved ones, and join in social get-togethers.

- **Welcoming exciting adventures:** Trying new things that excite us, like a new sport, exploring a fresh place, or diving into a creative project, is the need of the hour.

- **Let's rock our style:** Why not wear clothes that amp up our confidence and make us feel powerful? Let's try out vibrant colors, accessories, and styles that match our personality.

Rituals Honoring the Mother

- Pushing our physical limits with high-intensity workouts.

- Listing all the things we celebrate about ourselves.

- Indulging our senses with music, essential oils, dark chocolate, stylish clothes, or flowers.

- Wearing clothes that make us feel confident and feminine.

- Monitoring for signs of fertility and appreciating our amazing bodies.

- Cooking creatively by preparing a nourishing meal with seasonal ingredients, focusing on recipes that bring comfort and joy.

- Practicing gratitude each evening by writing down at least three things we're grateful for, focusing on the positive aspects of our life and the people who support us.

Autumn—Reflecting in the Harvest

The Witch's Wisdom

As the moon wanes, our energy turns inward and the Witch emerges. Linked to the waning moon and luteal phase (autumn/fall), this phase often brings PMS symptoms like headaches, mood swings, and irritability.

Women's emotions are sometimes dismissed as "just hormones," but it's more complex than that. Our struggles stem from suppressing our natural emotions. We battle our inner Wild Woman, longing to be seen and heard. She holds unique gifts, waiting to be shared. The Wild Woman urges us to face our pain and its roots. Only then can we truly heal, grow, and move forward.

In this phase, it's all about being kind to ourselves and realizing that slowing down can be just as powerful. Our bodies crave self-care, as they initially prepare each month as if we're pregnant, leading to a nesting instinct.

We're great at creating or organizing things during this time, like setting up new systems or cleaning out closets. This creative energy is also perfect for pursuing our dreams or getting creative with our business ideas. But if we don't channel this magical energy into something creative or fun—like painting, dancing, or cooking—what happens? It can build up and lead to outbursts of anger or tears.

In a cycle-focused life, we know that when this phase hits, we need some alone time. It's important to communicate this need to our family and make time for ourselves.

Activities and Celebrations

- **Making time for ourselves:** It's all about getting cozy and taking care of ourselves. Let's relax with a soothing bath using calming oils and dried roses. Roses have the highest frequency in nature, with rose essential oil vibrating at a rate of 320 MHz of electrical energy. This high vibrational frequency allows angels to connect more easily with roses (Hopler, 2019).

- **Reflecting and letting go:** Let's create a ritual to reflect and release any emotions or thoughts holding us back by having a releasing ceremony of sorts, being kind to ourselves, and taking it slow. For example, we can write down everything we want to let go of in our lives and burn this paper in a fire ceremony. Just using a candle and clay pot on our balcony would be enough. We can watch the fire burning all these things and transforming them into smoke.

- **Staying zen:** Let's try out stress-busting techniques like deep breathing, guided meditation, or using calming scents.

- **Eating mindfully:** Let's load up on magnesium-rich stuff like leafy greens, nuts, and seeds to help with mood swings and relaxation, and pick complex carbs to keep our energy stable.

- **Setting the scene:** Let's turn down the lights, play some soothing tunes, and fill the air with calming scents. This peaceful vibe can help ease any discomfort and bring some inner peace.

- **Easing into movement:** Trying restorative or Yin yoga, doing some easy stretches, or taking walks in nature are useful. These activities can help release tension and bring a sense of peace as our energy starts to wind down. Additionally, chanting is very powerful for women, especially because there is a direct correlation between the voice and our vagina through the vagus nerve. (In a female embryo, the vocal cords and ovaries are initially one organ that later splits into two as the embryo develops.) When we start chanting sacred sounds, we vibrate our whole body, and the sound we create aligns everything.

- **Artistic expression:** Let's engage in creative activities such as painting, drawing, or writing poetry to channel our inner emotions and artistic energy.

- **Mindful movement:** Participating in gentle activities like tai chi, qigong, and slow dancing helps us stay connected with our body and emotions.

Rituals Honoring the Enchantress

- Enjoying ample solitary time.

- Giving ourselves permission to cry and let our feelings flow freely.

- Practicing the art of saying no to commitments that don't serve our well-being.

- Performing a fire ceremony, which includes lighting candles, writing affirmations, and meditating under the moonlight.

Winter—Honoring the Retreat

The Wise Woman's Rest

The Wise Woman is the female archetype that focuses more on inner growth. Linked to the new moon and menstruation phase (winter), she's sometimes called the Crone, though the meaning of that term has shifted over time. In the past, "Crone" meant a wise older woman or leader. Now, it often brings up images of an old, worn-out woman.

The Wise Woman represents embracing the loss of fertility, beauty, and youth—things our society values in women. During menstruation, she calls on us to slow down and reflect. Our energy dips and we need more rest, but this phase brings renewal as our womb releases blood.

The dark moon marks the end of one phase, while the new moon starts a new one. If we've learned from our Wild Woman phase, all that wildness becomes wisdom. But we need to slow down, be patient, and let the wisdom unfold.

The Wise Woman doesn't fit society's expectations of women, so many of us keep her hidden away. However, she is deeply connected to the spiritual realm, offering us intuition and guidance as we transition into new phases of life.

During this time, we naturally slip into a meditative state, easily tapping into our inner wisdom and intuition. This builds a strong foundation to carry us through the end of the month as if we're floating on a cloud. It's a chance to let go of the past month's baggage and cleanse ourselves emotionally and physically.

Let's listen to our body's cues for rejuvenation and prioritize activities that nurture both our emotional and physical well-being.

Activities and Celebrations

- **Making time for meditation:** Incorporating meditation into our routine is ideal in this phase. Let's find a quiet spot, close our eyes, and try out a menstrual cycle meditation.

- **Opting for gentle movement or yoga:** We should honor our body's needs with gentle yoga or movement, focusing on stretches, restorative poses, or slow flows to ease any discomfort.

- **Sipping herbal teas:** Let's brew calming herbal teas like chamomile, red raspberry leaf, or ginger.

- **Indulging in self-care:** Let's enjoy restful activities that soothe both our body and our mind.

- **Creating a cozy sanctuary:** Why not make our space cozy with candles, soothing tunes, and comfy things, treating ourselves to a warm bath, leisurely reading, or just relaxing guilt-free?

- **Tuning into our bodies:** If we're tired, let's give ourselves permission to rest, using this time for relaxation.

- **Honoring the natural cycle:** Let's reconnect with ourselves and appreciate the beauty of renewal that our menstrual cycle brings, relaxing and indulging ourselves. Additionally, humming can help align the whole body and ease stagnation.

- **Vision or action boarding:** Let's create a vision board that we can act on in our upcoming cycle or year, focusing on our desires, intentions, passions, purpose, dreams, and aspirations.

- **Quiet time or silence:** Dedicating time to solitude and introspection allows us to rest and recharge without any guilt or pressure.

Rituals Honoring the Wise Woman

- Rocking something red.

- Taking moments to simply be, without any agenda.

- Figuring out where we want to focus our time, energy, and love in the upcoming cycle.

- Indulging in chocolate and comfort foods.

- Sacred bathing, taking a long, hot bath with Epsom salts, magnesium flakes, and essential oils like frankincense or sandalwood to soothe our body and mind.

- Practicing restorative yoga poses that encourage deep relaxation and healing.

Cultivating a Celebration Mindset

Every month, I gather with my closest friends to honor our cycles. We share stories, laugh, cry, and support each other. It's a powerful reminder of our collective strength. –Leah

Daily Practices to Honor Each Phase

A menstrual cycle journal helps us see what's working and what's not in our rituals. Through this, we can discover what brings us joy, comfort, and alignment in each phase. We can use this information to tweak our rituals and build a personalized tool kit.

Journaling regularly helps us dig deep into our thoughts and feelings. It especially helps us recognize which are thoughts and which are feelings. Thoughts come from our mind, creating stories, while feelings come from our heart, vibrating through our system. This practice gives us a better grip on our emotions so we can handle tough times with clarity and kindness.

With each new cycle, our journal transforms into a road map for personal growth. Documenting our experiences converts our journey into one of self-discovery and empowerment. In mysticism, every woman possesses a notebook known as the "Book of Shadows," where she meticulously records prayers, chants, herbs, cycles, recipes, and more, ensuring its legacy spans generations. By discerning patterns, refining rituals, and celebrating successes, we are not merely synchronizing with our cycle; we are harnessing our inherent power to effect change.

Champion the Maiden Archetype

- Be assertive by asking for what we want with calm confidence.

- Make plans and be social, surrounding ourselves with positivity and inspiration.

- Invest in self-growth by discovering our unique talents and celebrating our strengths.

- Dress to empower, wearing outfits that make us feel confident and active.

- Take a breather: Remember to pause and take a deep breath when needed.

Embody the Mother Archetype

- Prioritize self-care and spend time in nature.

- Clear out distractions and focus on what truly matters to us.

- Integrate into our local or online groups for support and belonging.

- Create and repeat affirmations that remind us of our strength, creativity, and independence.

- Take time to explore new places or ideas that spark our curiosity and excitement.

- Incorporate rituals like new moon ceremonies and gratitude practices into our lives.

Tap Into the Witch Archetype

- Experience and learn from all of our emotions.

- Spend time alone to connect with our inner self and create a sacred space for grounding.

- Protect our energy by establishing clear boundaries with others.

- Let go of past resentments and nurture forgiveness for ourselves and others. Writing about our emotions, dreams, and desires helps us better understand our inner self and release any built-up feelings.

● Treat ourselves to healing treatments to nurture ourselves.

● Spend time in nature, such as hiking, camping, or simply sitting outside, to ground ourselves and connect with the natural world.

Embrace the Wise Woman Archetype

● Rest during our bleeding days and harness the power of our menstrual cycle.

● Create new moon rituals to set intentions for our upcoming cycle.

● Slow down, meditate, journal, and connect with our inner wisdom through oracle readings.

● Let go of what no longer serves us.

● Embrace aging gracefully and share our wisdom with others as we continue to grow and evolve.

● Incorporate spiritual practices that resonate with us, such as prayer, meditation, or ritual work, to deepen our connection to our inner wisdom.

Mindfulness and Appreciation

Wondering about "mindful menstruation"? It's about understanding our whole cycle, not just the bleeding week. It helps us manage our emotional shifts and pain, increases our knowledge, improves our relationships, and helps us schedule better. Plus, it enhances our love and appreciation for our bodies.

We can start by tuning in when our period arrives and tracking how we feel throughout our cycle. It can take a few months to notice consistent patterns.

Mindful menstruation helps us embrace each phase's unique physical and emotional changes. Adjusting our yoga practice accordingly can improve our health and well-being.

It's about accepting and embracing our cycle without judgment. Understanding its impact on our relationships, body image, and motivation can empower us to live authentically.

Conclusion: A Continuous Cycle of Celebration

Periods reflect our well-being, reminding us of the connection between our body and our mind. Embracing our cycles means honoring nature's rhythms and welcoming this ceremony that happens in our lives every month. It's about living in sync with the universe, heeding our body's signals. This isn't just about challenging norms; it's about reclaiming ancestral wisdom.

Besides daily healthy eating and movement, celebrating our cycle means celebrating ourselves through each phase. This is about nurturing our closest relationship. When we pamper ourselves with joy and reverence, our life radiates feminine harmony.

Holistic cycle support starts with food, activities, and herbal remedies. We should trust our gut when picking what suits us best.

Our menstrual cycle ties us to the cosmos, reminding us of our natural place. Let's ditch shame and celebrate boldly. Let's start a love revolution for our period. When we celebrate it, we sync with life's cosmic beat.

This is our rallying cry: Let's love our period for its power, insight, and natural essence. By doing so, we reshape the narrative and pave the way for every woman to see her period as a source of strength, wisdom, and connection.

Chapter 9:
Creating Supportive Communities

The Power of Connection

People need connection and a sense of kinship, as we are all born with a longing to belong. Our communities (family, social circle, and friends) may provide much-needed support, especially during tough times, enhancing our emotional well-being. A supportive community, built on trust, helps us through challenges and celebrates our successes so we can all thrive.

Support and community are the lifeblood of our well-being, particularly for us women. Our sisterhood provides a sanctuary where we can share the joys and challenges of our menstrual cycle, celebrating each phase with understanding and compassion. The stigma around periods makes it even more important for us to have a caring family and community to lean on.

For most of us, our families—both immediate and extended—form our main support network. When we're young, our parents' understanding of our mood swings through different phases of our menstrual cycle, along with their guidance on how to track our own changes, is often all we need. As we grow older, we begin to need friends our own age with whom we can share our changes, cycles, and experiences. It's important to be open with our friends and the people in our circles. Practicing this openness helps us find the best ways to communicate and strengthens our support group over time. Understanding the importance of empathy and listening in building these connections allows us to provide the necessary support during emotional fluctuations.

Unfortunately, our parents or elders had their own life journeys, lived through different generations and times on Earth, and have their own stories. If our parents weren't taught about their cycles, they might not have passed this knowledge on to their children either. That's why it's imperative to build our own women circles, starting with you. Women thrive with other women. In shamanism, it's thought that women represent the water element, and when we come together and share, we clear our waters. In India, women have "peanut hours": Every afternoon, they meet to eat peanuts and share. These are the simplest ways to start building our own communities, allowing all of us to offload.

Building Women Circles

● **Start with one woman or acquaintance and build from there:** If there's someone in our life we like, they can be the beginning of our circle. We can reach out to a close friend, or an acquaintance with whom we share a deep bond, and invite her to create a sacred space where we can both share your menstrual journeys, supporting and uplifting each other.

● **Offer what you know:** Once we're part of a women circle, we can start inviting others. Things may take their time to grow, and we need to remember that we are doing this first and foremost for ourselves. Helping others builds a community for everyone, including us.

● **Join an existing circle:** There are unique women circles, such as yoni steam circles and tea or cacao ceremonies, taking place around the world, and we can easily search for and join one. It may be simpler to join a group that already exists rather than starting our own. By joining a group of like-minded women, attending their gatherings and events, and connecting with them on a deeper level, we help each other rise in our womanhood through the connections we start building.

- **Use social media to help build a community**: Utilizing platforms like Facebook, Meetup, and Twitter to create offline connections is another opportunity of this age. We can create an online gathering and invite our online friends to connect, discuss, and come together. Engaging in community activities like workshops or seminars can strengthen these bonds

Building a supportive women circle takes time, effort, and commitment. We have to be patient and allow it to develop gradually, letting the right people come together organically.

The Foundation of Community: Women Circles and Gatherings

Joining a women circle changed my life. The support, understanding, and love I found there helped me embrace my cycle and myself. –Ana

Women Circles: The Bedrock of Our Support Network

Our connection with other women and the feeling of belonging and welcome it provides is an integral part of our lives. The groups that we build with other women are with us through the ups and downs of our lives, our journeys, and our emotional shifts during the month, and they understand us better than anyone else. Whether we've cried, raged due to PMS, or withdrawn during our periods, our female friends and connections have always been there for us. This section will highlight why connecting with other women and building a circle is the cornerstone of our support system:

- **Showering us with unconditional love and acceptance:** These women gatherings offers us unconditional love and acceptance, no matter how moody we get. The unwavering love of other women gives us the confidence to talk openly about issues like heavy bleeding or cramps, without feeling ashamed.

- **Lending emotional support:** When we need emotional support, connecting with other women is usually the best thing we can do. They listen to our struggles, whether we're feeling overwhelmed (when our hormones dip) or inspired (during our ovulatory phase), and provide a safe, encouraging environment.

- **Acting as role models:** The women in our circles can be excellent role models. We learn how to handle life's challenges, including those related to our menstrual cycle, by observing the strength and resilience of other women in the group. Their experiences teach us to navigate difficult situations more effectively.

Women circles form the foundation of our support system. While no one is perfect, having a strong women circle support network helps us tackle life's challenges and embrace our womanhood with confidence. Encouraging open dialogue about menstrual health in these circles can demystify periods and reduce stigma.

Strengthening Bonds

Here are some strategies to strengthen bonds within women circles and gatherings, specifically centered around women's menstrual cycles:

- **Communicate openly about menstrual health with heartfelt honesty:** Sharing our menstrual experiences and needs with open hearts within our women circle is important to feel heard and understood. Let the circle be a place where we feel deeply heard and recognized, cultivating empathy. Open communication helps avoid misunderstandings and fosters empathy.

- **Show appreciation and gratitude:** Whether it's a member who comforts us during an emotional breakthrough or a friend who offers a listening ear, acknowledging and thanking those who support us during our cycle can strengthen our relationships and create mutual respect.

- **Be there for each other:** Being there for each other during challenging times and our menstrual cycles, offering a listening ear, comfort, and help with tasks when needed, shows that we care about each other's well-being. Reliability builds trust and support.

- **Set boundaries:** While supporting each other is imperative, setting boundaries is equally vital. Clearly communicating our needs and limits regarding our menstrual health ensures that everyone's comfort levels are maintained.

- **Work through challenges together:** Approaching menstrual-related challenges (both physical and emotional) as a team strengthens our bond. For this to happen, we have to be open to feedback, apologize when necessary, and find solutions together.

Scheduling regular meetings or events can keep the connection strong and provide consistent support. Building and maintaining strong relationships within women circles, especially around menstrual health, requires effort, communication, and a willingness to support each other.

Building Your Extended Community

Starting Small

Women circles are gatherings of women with shared interests or goals. They can be formal meetings, meetups in parks, monthly mother gatherings, or spontaneous get-togethers in someone's home. These circles can provide social support, mutual aid, and shared experiences, helping members feel a sense of belonging. In this section, we'll look at how we women can create and manage our own women circles that cater to our needs and the challenges we encounter.

Setting Up and Managing a Women's Community Group for Menstrual Health: Nurture the Organic Growth of Your Circle

Let's begin by inviting a few close friends to gather in a cozy, welcoming space. Share stories, experiences, and rituals that honor our sisterhood and our menstrual health, allowing the circle to grow naturally through personal connections:

- **Evaluate the need:** Look into existing groups to see what is already available, such as local meetups, social media groups, or community gatherings. Consider partnering with them, or reflect on whether starting a new circle is necessary and what doing so could offer.

- **Find our niche:** Identifying our specific area of interest is the first step. Our niche could encompass menstrual health, mental well-being, parenting, personal growth, meditation, or any other shared experiences. This will help define our group's purpose and attract like-minded members. We should ask ourselves:

○ What aspects of menstrual health are we passionate about?

○ What challenges in this area do we want to address?

○ What outcomes do we hope to achieve?

○ Who do we seek to connect with?

○ How can our group stand out and be a safe space for women to offload?

● **Form the core team:** You are the core team; yet, if you feel you need help, start with a small team to share responsibilities. This will ensure specific invitations are sent on time, locations are chosen wisely, and, if there are objects involved (e.g., yoga mats, candles, or print outs), they are organized in advance.

● **Choose a meeting place:** Initially, it's better to select free, convenient locations such as community centers, parks, or someone's home.

● **Choose our platform:** We have to select a tool or service to host and manage our circle. Options include websites, social media, forums, or chat apps. It can be as easy as starting a Telegram or WhatsApp group. Consider:

○ necessary features (e.g., event creation, polls, blogs)

○ member preferences (e.g., ease of use, mobile-friendly)

○ pros and cons of each platform

● **Ensure long-term success:** Successful women circles rely on clear goals, teamwork, and passionate members. A strong core team allows the circle to focus on its mission and make the most of its resources (Edelman, 2012).

Nurturing Engagement Within and Beyond—Inviting Members to Our Circle

The final step in creating a women circle is to invite members who will join, participate, and contribute. These members can be friends, family, colleagues, or anyone passionate about supporting and uplifting each other. Inviting members is crucial for the growth and sustainability of your circle. Here are some strategies to attract members:

● **Word of mouth:** Start by sharing the idea with close friends and family. Personal invitations are powerful and help create a close-knit community from the start.

● **Personal invitations:** Invite women you know personally who might benefit from and contribute to the circle. Share your vision and the purpose of the gatherings.

● **Sharing in existing groups:** Mention your women circle in other groups or gatherings you are part of, like book clubs, parenting groups, or yoga classes. This can help you reach women who are already interested in community and support.

● **Creating a welcoming environment:** Emphasize that the circle is a safe space for sharing, support, and growth. Make sure new members know they are joining a nurturing and nonjudgmental environment.

• **Using social media:** Share your women circle on your social media profiles. Highlight the sense of community, support, and shared experiences. Use stories and posts to show what the circle is about and how it benefits its members.

• **Hosting open gatherings:** Occasionally, host open gatherings where potential new members can experience the circle. This can be a great way for women to see the value and decide to join.

• **Encouraging referrals:** We can ask existing members to invite or recommend our circle to their friends or family members who might be interested. Personal recommendations can help attract women who are a good fit for the circle.

Fostering Open Communication

Create a Judgment-Free Haven

Encouraging open and compassionate conversations about menstrual health in women circles is the way forward. Let every member feel safe to share their story, knowing they will be met with kindness and understanding. Here's how to do it:

• **Create a safe environment:** We should ensure everyone feels comfortable discussing menstrual health without judgment. Honesty and openness are key.

• **Listen actively:** Everyone should pay attention to what each member is saying about their menstrual experiences. We should respect their views and ask open-ended questions to promote sharing.

- **Practice empathy:** Everyone should understand and validate their feelings about menstrual health, even if some of us may have different experiences and opinions. Showing support and understanding is crucial.

- **Schedule regular gatherings:** We should plan regular activities such as meetups, tea sessions, coffee dates, meditation mornings, or group walks to create opportunities for open communication without distractions.

- **Apologize and forgive:** Members must resolve conflicts with apologies and forgiveness to maintain an environment of trust and respect. This helps our circle to remain a supportive and nurturing space

Organizing Community Activities—Hosting Heart-Centered Women's Gatherings

Women circle events are powerful tools for promoting positive change. By organizing storytelling sessions, communal rituals, and sharing circles, we celebrate the beauty of womanhood. Integrating cultural and heritage practices to deepen the connection and support within the community is priceless.

Menstrual Hygiene Awareness Campaigns

We can host events to educate the community about menstrual hygiene. Examples include:

- **Workshops and seminars:** Inviting health professionals to talk about menstrual hygiene management.

- **School programs:** Conducting sessions in schools to educate both boys and girls about menstruation, breaking stereotypes and taboos.

Free Distribution of Period Products

Let's ensure menstrual equity by organizing donation drives for period products. This can also allow us to do some research about the different products and understand more about what we use and their effects. For instance:

- **Community donation drives:** Collecting and distributing menstrual products to those in need.

- **Partnerships with local businesses:** Collaborating with shops and pharmacies to provide free or discounted period products.

Awareness Campaigns

Raising awareness about menstrual health through various community events might include:

- **Public lectures and panels:** Discussing menstrual health issues, rights, and gender equality.

- **Social media campaigns:** Using platforms to spread information and destigmatize menstruation.

Cultural and Heritage Celebrations

Let's integrate menstrual health education into cultural events through:

- **Heritage celebrations:** Highlighting historical practices and modern advances in menstrual health.

- **Community festivals:** Including booths or segments dedicated to menstrual health awareness.

Skill Development and Training

We can promote overall wellness by incorporating menstrual health into broader health initiatives:

- **Yoga and meditation classes**: Including information on how movement impacts menstrual health.

- **Health and wellness workshops:** Offering classes on nutrition and lifestyle choices that support menstrual health.

Leveraging Technology—Digital Tools for Connectivity

Let's use social media and virtual platforms to build a supportive online community. We can host regular virtual gatherings where women can share their experiences and support each other through their menstrual journeys.

- **Virtual awareness campaigns:** We can use social media platforms like Facebook, Instagram, and TikTok to raise awareness about important topics such as menstrual hygiene, mental health, self-care, and empowerment. Share educational content, host live Q&A sessions with experts, and debunk myths about menstruation.

- **Online donation drives for free period products:** Platforms like GoFundMe or local community groups on

Facebook can be used to gather donations for various causes, such as providing period products, supporting women's shelters, or funding educational programs.

● **Digital educational programs in schools:** Collaborating with schools by using video conferencing tools like Zoom or Microsoft Teams can allow us to provide educational sessions on a range of topics, ensuring comprehensive education for all students.

● **Social media engagement:** We can engage with our community through regular posts and interactive content, sharing stories, tips, and personal experiences and information on various aspects of women's lives, building a supportive online community.

● **Virtual support groups:** Let's create online support groups on platforms like Telegram, WhatsApp, and Facebook. These provide a safe space for women to share their experiences and seek advice on a variety of issues, from menstrual health to mental well-being and personal growth.

● **Hosting virtual events:** We can organize virtual events such as webinars, panel discussions, and live streams focusing on diverse topics relevant to women circles, including health, wellness, empowerment, and community building.

● **Sharing resources and information:** Utilizing social networks to share valuable resources is a good idea. We can post links to informative articles, videos, and infographics on a wide range of topics, from menstrual health to self-care and empowerment, on social media platforms (Kacane & Hernàndez-Serrano, 2023).

Overcoming Challenges—Resolve Conflicts With Compassion

Our need to feel empowered is linked to how we handle issues within women circles and gatherings. For this, we need to focus on the importance of good communication and resolving conflicts. These skills are imperative for creating supportive spaces where women can feel empowered during their periods.

Conflicts often happen when people have different opinions or misunderstand each other. If these conflicts aren't handled well, they can cause stress and harm relationships. While it's normal to disagree, ongoing conflict is damaging. Being heard and hearing the other person helps reduce tension and leads to peaceful solutions. This means negotiating, calming down before talking, focusing on solving the problem, and respecting each other's views.

Listening calmly and without interrupting helps avoid misunderstandings and keeps conflicts from getting worse. Working together to find solutions involves everyone suggesting ideas, being willing to compromise, and sticking to the agreed solution.

By using these conflict resolution skills, women circles can create supportive environments throughout life and its challenges. This support is necessary for women to feel confident and empowered, especially during their menstrual cycles and in women circles. Empowerment is closely tied to how well we understand and support each other.

Conflict Resolution Strategies

Creating a harmonious environment is necessary for our empowerment and growth, as conflicts can disrupt the harmony in communities. To resolve conflicts and ensure a harmonious gathering:

- **Let's acknowledge the conflict:** Ignoring conflicts can make them worse. It's better to recognize and address issues promptly.

- **Let's define the problem**: Clearly identifying the cause of the conflict is important. Both parties need to agree on the issue and discuss unmet needs.

- **Let everyone have a say:** We must ensure that each party in the conflict has an equal chance to express their views. A positive, respectful dialogue with set ground rules should take place.

- **Let's agree on a solution:** We have to investigate the issue thoroughly before deciding on a resolution. We need to look for underlying causes and understand all perspectives.

- **Let's determine roles in the solution:** Both sides should feel the solution is fair. Through open dialogue, each party should understand and accept their role in resolving the conflict.

Evaluating Effectiveness

Effective circles and gatherings with women and communities play a vital role in our individual and collective well-being, which can empower women during their menstrual cycles.

Techniques to Reflect on Emotional Well-Being

- **Subjective assessment of our well-being:** It's important to understand how we feel about our own lives, including aspects like our relationships, family, friend circles, career, stress levels, health and diet, the planet, and how they are affected during the phases of our cycle. Do we feel satisfied? And does this change when we have PMS? Can we use these changes as a sign to discuss and go deeper in these areas within ourselves? Subjective assessment is crucial.

- **Subjective assessment of collective living:** Assessing how we feel about collective aspects of our community such as safety and social trust within the space is essential. These factors influence how supportive and empowering a women's group can be.

- **Community well-being as a whole:** Beyond our own assessments, understanding the well-being of our circle involves looking at cohesion, shared values, and a sense of belonging. This collective well-being captures how well people live together and support one another.

By combining objective data (like economic indicators) with subjective assessments (our feelings about our lives and community), we can get a comprehensive view of our well-being. This approach helps us design better projects and services that respond to the needs of both individuals and the community.

Conclusion: A Continuous Journey

Building strong connections within our women circles and communities brings many benefits. These supportive networks help us through tough times and improve our emotional well-being. By putting in effort to strengthen these bonds, we enjoy long-term rewards like better decision-making and more vibrant communities. Engaging with our community creates a sense of belonging and empowers us, making our neighborhoods more livable and connected.

Sisterhood is vital for women, providing a unique support system that understands and uplifts us. Women's groups are necessary for fostering this sisterhood, and it's easy to start one yourself. When we focus on nurturing these relationships, we not only support each other better but also build a stronger, more inclusive society. Investing in our immediate and extended communities ensures we all thrive together.

Chapter 10:
We Are in This Together

The Universal Nature of Menstrual Experience

Around half of the world's population either has experienced in the past or is still experiencing menstruation monthly, yet many people don't understand its emotional impact and are still not talking about it. Menstrual health is indispensable for our overall well-being, affecting our physical, mental, and social health from our very first period to menopause.

Those around us need to understand more about the impact of our periods and how their challenges affect our lives. Both men and women should embrace this reality—the truth of our existence—and use the opportunity for growth to better manage our lives. Men often learn about menstruation through personal relationships. Expanding their understanding can foster greater empathy and support.

Menstruation affects everyone:

- **Women:** We directly deal with the physical and emotional challenges of our period.

- **Family members:** Our family notice changes in our moods and activities.

- **Work and school:** Menstruation can affect attendance and performance, so supportive environments are essential.

- **Community:** Issues like mood shifts may impact our attendance or performance at community activities.

Seeing menstruation as a shared experience helps build empathy and support. By understanding its impact, we can all work toward a better-integrated lifestyle.

This chapter aims to promote understanding, support, and unity in addressing menstruation as a global issue. Recognizing menstruation as a natural part of life can help break down the stigma and taboos often associated with it. This chapter also highlights the importance of empathy and support for us menstruating women, acknowledging the physical and emotional challenges we face. The aim is to educate about the biological, emotional, and social aspects of menstruation to encourage informed discussions.

Understanding the Impact on All

Direct Impact

Every month, menstruation brings to us a mix of physical and emotional symptoms like cramps, headaches, mood swings, and stress, and for most women, it also brings a need to hide. Understanding these changes helps us understand ourselves better, which directly impacts our engagement with the external world.

Hormonal changes before and during periods cause ups and downs—and especially lots of downs. Some days we feel great, while other days we feel tired and irritable. For some, these changes bring energy and creativity, but for others, they cause bloating, headaches, and fatigue. Menstrual disorders, like heavy bleeding and pelvic pain, can disrupt our daily life, making us miss commitments and affecting our mental health.

Sadly, we don't talk enough about menstrual health. Terms like PMS and premenstrual dysphoric disorder (PMDD) can make normal changes sound like illnesses, reinforcing unfair stereotypes.

Two common misconceptions harm women. One is that all women have negative mood changes during their period, leading to outdated beliefs that women can't handle certain jobs. The other is that menstruation has no biological impact, ignoring our very real struggles and hindering research.

Premenstrual symptoms are hormone-based but also influenced by social and psychological factors. While research often highlights negatives, we should also recognize the benefits of our hormonal changes. Instead of suppressing our natural cycles with synthetic hormones at the first sign of hormonal imbalance, we should focus on how diet, exercise, and stress management can help balance hormones naturally.

Menstruation also involves social attitudes and stigma, which can cause stress and shame. We need to find the courage to start the conversation and openly discuss our experiences so that, with each step we take, we get closer to normalizing period talk and breaking down this stigma.

Indirect Impact

Menstruation doesn't just affect those who experience it directly; it also impacts the people around them. Men in families or communities, for example, are indirectly affected by the hormonal changes and mood swings of those who menstruate. Understanding these experiences is key to offering the right support.

Menstruation affects family dynamics and relationships. Parents, siblings, partners, and friends are often not equipped to handle the changes. For partners, the monthly cycle can bring recurring stress, impacting relationship satisfaction. The anticipation and experience of premenstrual symptoms can be exhausting for both the person experiencing them and their partner. Open communication and understanding are crucial in these situations.

Couples often report lower satisfaction and well-being during their partner's cycle, highlighting the need for better understanding and support. Not only can men improve their partner's experience by learning about PMS and PMDD and providing appropriate support, but they can also enhance relationship satisfaction.

Work colleagues are also indirectly affected by menstruation. Many women feel unable to tell their managers about menstrual-related absences due to fear of trivialization or embarrassment. Building an open and inclusive workplace culture can help normalize menstruation. Providing information, resources, and training for management teams on periods and their effect on all can foster a supportive environment.

Let's break down the stigma and educate those around us—partners, colleagues, friends, and family members—about our periods. Finding simple resources to share information can make menstruation a more accepted and understood topic, just like many other subjects that were once taboo.

Building Empathy and Understanding

Education for Everyone

Periods, which many people feel awkward talking about, actually affect society a lot. There are many rules and taboos around periods. Many of us often try to hide them, which can change how families and relationships work.

The lack of open discussion about periods leaves young girls in the dark about this natural process. Even when they ask questions, most of the time adults avoid talking about it because they feel awkward due to cultural or religious beliefs. As a result, most young girls are never properly initiated into this new chapter of their life, which means they miss out on important information about their bodily changes and how to handle themselves and their health during their periods. Most mothers, unfortunately, only talk about the products we should use and how no one should know about our periods, instead of talking about cycles, mood shifts, emotions, well-being, diet, and more. This keeps the taboo around bleeding alive.

Recognition brings clarity. Periods and their effects should be acknowledged to make the topic feel lighter and less burdensome. As menstruation is often seen as a taboo, many young people go through life never learning how to handle their needs around the topic of periods. If we all step into a new reality of normalizing what is already very normal and natural, this pink elephant in the middle of the room will disappear.

Despite its universal nature, menstruation is rarely openly discussed among males. However, their involvement is essential in supporting women—men's partners, sisters, mothers, and daughters—in menstrual cycle management and breaking down societal taboos. We need men who are ready to hold space for women to bleed freely and acknowledge the power of this time. In some cultures, women are advised to marry men who have sisters, as mothers believe that these men already understand the emotional shifts of a woman and can handle them better than others. Making this a reality for us all is a matter of intention and education.

Having access to menstrual hygiene products, knowing how to choose them, and educating ourselves about them is essential for preventing the health risks associated with poor menstrual management. By promoting open and factual discussions about menstruation, education can challenge societal taboos and promote a more inclusive and supportive environment for us all.

Sharing Stories

Stories and personal narratives are powerful tools for understanding the experiences of young people and women, and for talking openly about sensitive topics like periods. Unfortunately, period stories are not often shared and many of us feel embarrassed to discuss our period and the period journey openly, even though it's a natural part of life.

This discomfort can lead to delayed care and unnecessary suffering, especially for those dealing with heavy bleeding or pain. By encouraging conversations about periods, we can create a supportive community that hears, understands, and guides us through the challenges.

The negative talk around periods, focusing only on sharing stories of pain, discomfort, moodiness, is linked to the stigma around the topic. Due to cultural taboos, some of us feel that we can only talk about our periods by complaining. However, as long as the discussions around menstruation stay negative, they reinforce the stigma. Instead, we should encourage each other to talk about periods in a completely different way. Rather than keeping our periods hidden and playing into a system that oppresses women, we can welcome our period each month and monitor our symptoms, the color of our blood, the heaviness of our flow, and the changes in our bodies. By recognizing that our bodies are still capable of bringing new life into the world, we can share this with our circles to transform oppression into freedom.

Every voice has its place and all women deserve to be heard. Let's amplify these conversations and ensure that all of us women receive the acknowledgment we deserve.

Practical Support Systems

In Homes and Families

Family support is imperative, not just for managing the physical aspects of periods with confidence, but also for navigating a world that often stigmatizes this natural bodily function.

Tips for Creating Supportive Environments at Home for Managing Periods Comfortably

- **Talking openly:** We should discuss menstruation openly at home with our families to make it a normal topic.

- **Empowering with knowledge:** We should feel confident enough around our family, or practice so we can develop this confidence, to inform them about our period—and eliminate shame for all of us.

- **Family support:** Our family environment is the centerpiece for practicing transparency in sharing our journey. Families can play a big role by encouraging good hygiene practices and supporting us.

- **Combating stigma:** Family support boosts our confidence so that we fight against the stigma and discrimination related to menstruation, making us feel more comfortable.

- **Positive communication:** Open and positive conversations within families and among peers can improve attitudes toward our period.

- **Financial help:** Providing free access to sanitary pads increases confidence in managing periods comfortably at home.

In Workplaces

In workplaces, how we deal with menstruation will vary depending on our roles. The differences in our roles can influence how easily we are able to manage our schedules, with some positions offering more flexibility than others. Many of us never discuss anything period related at work, often attributing any absence to general illness. This secrecy makes things hard for many of us to manage our symptoms and go ahead with day-to-day life like nothing is happening. This makes us feel pressured to follow unwritten rules about how to behave when menstruating, even though we find these rules outdated.

These challenges reflect broader societal attitudes toward menstruation, and many workplaces lack specific policies to support employees with menstrual health issues. Surprisingly, most employers don't offer any support in this regard. However, creating a supportive workplace environment can make a big difference. It can help us female employees feel seen, valued, respected, and understood, leading to better attendance and performance.

Simple things can change our whole experience in the workplace. Employers can create a work culture that respects menstrual health and provides necessary accommodations. This might include flexible schedules, remote working, access to period products, and paid leave for medical appointments related to menstrual health. These simple but powerful steps would build an inclusive and supportive workplace for everyone.

Celebrating Togetherness

Cultural Festivals From Around the World That Honor Menstruation

Periods can be uncomfortable, but it's worse when they're not celebrated by the community. Many of us deal with them silently, feeling guilty for wanting to rest and eat comfort foods. We often avoid friends and family to prevent our mood swings from affecting others.

Some face even tougher challenges as a result of conditions like PMDD, PCOS, or endometriosis, enduring severe pain but still pushing through daily responsibilities.

We need to change how we view periods. Instead of seeing them as obstacles, we should listen to our bodies and work at a comfortable pace. In some cultures, menstruation is honored and celebrated, and this idea should be more widespread.

Different cultures have unique menstrual rituals. Here are four fascinating examples:

- **Ojibwe (American Midwest):** Ojibwe women traditionally isolate themselves in a moon lodge during menstruation to cleanse and recharge. They avoid sex, ceremonies, and food preparation and are relieved from childcare duties. Other women visit them and bring them meals, strengthening community bonds.

- **Assam (India):** During the monsoon season, temples in Assam close for four days as the goddess Kamakhya is believed to be menstruating. This period is marked by the *Ambubachi Mela* festival, where people celebrate and seek blessings. When the temple reopens, devotees receive wet cloths symbolizing the goddess's menstrual fluid, believed to bring good fortune.

- **Tikuna Tribe (Brazil):** When a Tikuna girl has her first period, she lives alone for a year, visited only by her grandmother, who teaches her traditional skills. After this period, a ceremony called *Pelazón*, involving three days of rituals, dances, and feasts, marks her transition into womanhood.

- **Hupa Tribe (California):** The Hupa Tribe celebrates a girl's first period with the Flower Dance, or *Ch'ilwa:l*, lasting several days. The girl wears a blue jay-feather face covering while the community participates in traditional songs and dances. The celebration ends with a large feast and elaborate gifts (Aquino, 2020).

These traditions show how different cultures honor menstruation, turning it into a time of rest, learning, and community bonding.

Creating New Traditions to Recognize and Support

Menstruation

In today's fast-paced world, we've lost touch with many traditional rituals, leaving us feeling exhausted. However, we can create new ways to honor menstruation, a natural and significant part of our lives. Here are some ideas:

- Why not light aromatic candles and incense, creating a cozy atmosphere for practicing gentle yoga or meditation during our period?

- Chanting is another powerful way to connect our vocal cords and yoni due to the link between our voice and our vagina through the vagus nerve, as discussed in Chapter 8. When we chant, we align our bodies with the healing vibrations of sound and vibrate the vagus nerve, creating a connection from throat to root.

- Gathering fresh flowers for a warm bubble bath or hosting a gathering of menstruating friends for reflection and rejuvenation are also wonderful ideas.

A ceremony to celebrate the initiation into womanhood can be simple and flexible, whether in person or virtual. It can involve just one adult and the young person, or could include friends and family. Here are a few ideas to make it unique:

- **Blessings:** We can speak or write intentions for the young person. These can be simple heartfelt wishes for their growth and the qualities we admire in them. We can share these aloud and encourage others to do the same. The young person can also share their own intentions and dreams for the future.

- **Rituals:** Incorporate simple actions to connect with each other and the moment through natural elements:

  ○ **Fire:** Light a candle to start the ceremony and put out the candle flame properly with a wick dipper to close the ceremony (remember, candles have a very strong power and influence in many rituals, and they should be put out—not blown out).

  ○ **Water:** Brew a special herbal tea while speaking blessings, then drink it together—possibly offering some to the Earth as well.

  ○ **Earth:** Sharing food like raspberries or red candies to honor the menstrual cycle while connecting through plants.

  ○ **Air:** Giving a meaningful gift, like roses or a hand-me-down that can be treasured (Rabins, n.d.).

Additional ideas include presenting flowers or drawing a bubble bath with candles to let the young person relax afterward. These new traditions give us a chance to learn to nurture ourselves. This time of nurturing reconnects us with a deeper layer of our essence.

Conclusion: A Call to Collective Action

When we talk openly about menstruation, we break down barriers and build bridges of understanding and empathy. It's a journey we must all take together. –Michael

Understanding that we are all interconnected in the journey of menstruation can help us focus on inner work to address period-related stigma and emotional shifts. Here are key areas to consider:

● Firstly, embracing open discussions about our menstrual experiences helps break down internalized stigma and creates a supportive environment. Sharing our stories and challenges can empower us and those around us to view periods as a natural and important aspect of life for all of us.

● Secondly, it's essential to build our own confidence and skills to talk about menstrual health openly. Educating ourselves and the people around us and in our circles can help break the silence and reduce the shame often associated with periods.

● Thirdly, advocating for our own menstrual health means recognizing and honoring our bodies' needs. By practicing self-care and seeking support when needed, we can manage our menstrual health with dignity and confidence.

● Lastly, creating supportive spaces in our homes, workplaces, and communities can help us connect with other women and share our experiences and period-related topics with greater ease.

By focusing on these practices and aspects of inner work, we can transform our relationship with other women and menstruation, embracing it as a normal, supported part of our lives.

Conclusion

Celebrating Our Collective Journey

Just as we began this journey by recognizing the profound unspoken bond that menstruation creates among women, we now come full circle. This book has been a celebration of that bond, an invitation to honor the natural rhythms of our bodies and embrace the power that lies within us.

Each of the four phases of the menstrual cycle brings unique physical, psychological, and emotional changes. By reconnecting with these ancient rhythms, we can harness their true nature and inner strength.

Interestingly, the menstrual cycle inspired the measurement of the month, aligning with the lunar cycle. The phases of the moon symbolize different energetic states in the menstrual cycle: the Maiden, the Mother, the Witch, and the Wise Woman.

Our menstrual cycle affects everything from our appetite to our sleep patterns to our moods. Cycle syncing—adapting our eating and exercise habits to our menstrual phases—can be a powerful tool. Tracking our cycle helps us identify trends, allowing us to develop habits that support our needs in each stage.

Through our shared exploration, we've explored the intricate dance of our menstrual cycle, understanding the deep connections to ancient wisdom and modern science. By embracing this knowledge, we can not only better understand and support our natural rhythms, enhancing our overall health and well-being, but also practice being more present and available for ourselves—a reflection of our inner strength, resilience, and capacity for growth.

Recognizing Our Shared Strength

In recent years, people have started to see our menstrual cycle in a new light. Instead of viewing it as a hassle, there's a growing understanding that working with our body's natural rhythms can boost productivity, improve self-care, and make us feel more empowered.

Period-tracking apps help us track our periods, symptoms, and fertility. They also offer insights into different cycle phases and give us tips for how we should adjust our exercise, self-care, and work routines. These apps help us align our activities with our cycles, improving both our physical and our emotional health.

Using technology to track our cycles changes the way we think about periods—from something to be ashamed of to a source of strength. Embracing our menstrual cycles helps us connect with our bodies, build resilience, and strengthen our circles and community. Understanding our bodies is a powerful way to empower ourselves and support each other.

Empowering Ourselves and Others

Taking care of our menstrual health is an essential part of overall well being. Here are some steps we can take to embrace and promote menstrual health:

- **Understand our bodies:** Let's learn about the biological aspects of our menstrual cycle. Understanding how our body works during this time can help us better manage symptoms and know when to act and when not during the month.

- **Practice self-care:** Let's engage in self-care practices to nurture our emotional well-being during our cycle. Relaxation exercises, meditation, journaling, or expressing our emotions can help alleviate stress, anxiety, and mood swings.

● **Seek support:** Let's create a supportive environment for ourselves and seek emotional support from our loved ones. Sometimes, just a big, deep-felt hug can help us feel understood and supported.

● **Promote menstrual hygiene:** Let's promote good menstrual hygiene practices, such as using clean menstrual products and changing them regularly. This helps prevent infections and maintains our overall health.

● **Manage symptoms:** Let's find ways to manage menstrual symptoms that may affect our daily life. Whether it's through nutrition, exercise, or other lifestyle changes, we should take proactive steps.

● **Challenge stigma:** Let's challenge the stigma surrounding period talk by educating others on the importance of menstrual health. By openly discussing and normalizing the topic, we can break down barriers and create a more transparent environment for everyone.

● **Embrace the cycle:** Embracing our periods is about more than just understanding its biological aspects. It's about recognizing the importance of menstrual health and well-being in our life.

Envisioning a Supportive Future

Imagine a future where menstrual health is openly supported, celebrated, and seamlessly integrated into every aspect of life. In this world, everyone, regardless of gender, plays an active role in supporting menstrual health, creating a community where period dignity is a given.

With period dignity, we will all have access to menstrual products, accurate information about menstrual health, and clean, private facilities for managing our periods. We will be free from the shame and embarrassment often associated with menstruation. Period dignity will be recognized as a matter of human rights and equality.

Owning our period and embracing all of its phases and archetypes connects us with our inner sacred feminine. Embracing these archetypes help us realize our unique strengths and enhances our empowerment and self-awareness, making period dignity a reality for everyone.

Picture a world where menstruation is no longer a barrier to education, health, or opportunities. Through social change, we can create a future where our cycle and our womanhood are celebrated and integrated into all aspects of life.

Gratitude and a Rallying Cry

Thank you. This book is a testament to the strength of our collective sisterhood. It serves as a reminder that we are never alone in our experiences. The solidarity we share is a source of immense power, capable of breaking down stigma and creating a culture of understanding, connection, guidance, and support.

As you close this book, remember that the journey does not end here. The knowledge and insights gained are tools to be carried forward, shared with others, and integrated into daily life. By aligning our routines with our natural cycles, we nurture ourselves, deepen our relationships, live more authentically, and are more real in life.

Together, let's continue to honor the sacred ceremony of our bodies, celebrate our innate power, and support each other in every phase of life. This is not just about menstruation; it's about embracing every aspect of womanhood with grace, confidence, and unwavering strength within a heartbeat, and seeing ourselves reflected in the eyes of all other women.

Thank you for joining me on this journey. May we all continue to thrive, hand in hand, heart to heart, empowered by the shared experience of our cycle and the unbreakable bond of sisterhood and unity. This book has been woven from my personal journey of discovering and embracing the rhythms of my own menstrual cycle. May it inspire you to start your own path of empowerment, finding strength and solidarity in the shared tapestry of our experiences as women.

References

Aiyana, S. (2017, September 9). *The 4 seasons of a woman's cycle explained week by week.* Rising Woman. https://risingwoman.com/4-archetypes-of-the-female-cycle/

Aquino, L. (2020, October 23). *5 menstrual rituals around the world & what they can teach us.* The Fornix. https://blog.flexfits.com/menstrual-rituals-around-the-world/

An Ayurvedic approach to a healthy cycle. (2024). Banyan Botanicals. https://www.banyanbotanicals.com/info/ayurvedic-living/living-ayurveda/health-guides/healthy-cycle-guide/

Beyk, E. (2021, June 10).*The lost knowledge of the creative power of the womb.* Erika Mohssen Beyk. https://erikamohssen-beyk.com/nature-natural-health-and-food/the-lost-knowledge-of-the-creative-power-of-the-womb/

Boga, S. (n.d.). *The importance of healing your womb.* Kimiya Healing. https://www.kimiyahealing.co.uk/post/unlocking-your-female-energy-through-the-womb-space

Brown, D. (2021, July 30). *How can PMS affect your relationships?* Psychology Central. https://psychcentral.com/blog/pms-relationships

Building a supportive network of family and friends. (n.d.). Health Hub. https://www.healthhub.sg/live-healthy/buildingasupportivenetwork

Burke, S. (2023). Wisdom from the elders: Kinship care that honours traditional Indigenous ways. *AlterNative: An International Journal of Indigenous Peoples*, *19*(3), 635–645. https://doi.org/10.1177/11771801231189842

Community action to overcome menstrual hygiene taboos. (2024, January 2). Global Waters. https://www.globalwaters.org/resources/assets/community-action-overcome-menstrual-hygiene-taboos

Community groups: how to create and facilitate community groups. (2024, April 7). Faster Capital. https://fastercapital.com/content/Community-groups—How-to-create-and-facilitate-community-groups.html

Couto-Ferreira, M. E. & Verderame, L. (2018). *Cultural constructions of the uterus in pre-modern societies, past and present.* Cambridge Scholar Publishing.

Culbertson, Z. (n.d.). *Meditations to optimize your cycle.* Circle Bloom. https://circlebloom.com/meditations-to-optimize-your-cycle/

Dorwart, L. (2023, May 30). *Everything you need to know about cycle syncing.* Health. https://www.health.com/cycle-syncing-7500732

Edelman, C. (2012, April 3). *Developing a supportive community.* Cindy Black-Edelman. https://blank-edelman.com/blog/2012/04/developing-a-supportive-community-for-yourself/

Edi. (2023, June 18). *How to use rituals for a better menstrual cycle.* Wellness With Edie. https://wellnesswithedie.com/menstrual-cycle-rituals/

The Editors of Encyclopaedia Britannica. (2024, January 20). *Uterus.* Encyclopedia Britannica. https://www.britannica.com/science/uterus

8 ways you can support your partner during that time of the month. (n.d.). Livia. https://mylivia.com/blogs/news/8-ways-you-can-support-your-partner-during-that-time-of-the-month

Ezrin, S. (2022, February 24). *A comprehensive guide to sun salutation sequences A, B, and C.* Healthline. https://www.healthline.com/health/fitness/sun-salutation-sequence

Family conflict. (2014, August 21). Better Health Channel. https://www.betterhealth.vic.gov.au/health/healthyliving/family-conflict

The 5 best period tracking apps of 2024. (2024, March 21). FemTech World. https://www.femtechworld.co.uk/special/the-5-best-period-tracking-apps-of-2024/

The follicular phase: Renewal and vitality. (n.d.). Period Shop. https://periodshop.com.au/blogs/all/embracing-the-follicular-phase-nurturing-renewal-and-vitality

The four seasons of your cycle. (2022, April 7). Cycle. https://cycle.care/en/de-vier-seizoenen-van-je-cyclus

Gooding, J. T. (n.d.). *Womb energy is so important for mothers and mothers-to-be – Diana Beaulieu Interview.* No Mum Is An Island. https://nomumisanisland.com/womb-energy/

Herrity, J. (2024, April 9). *5 conflict resolution strategies: Steps, benefits and tips.* Indeed. https://www.indeed.com/career-advice/career-development/conflict-resolution-strategies

The hidden link: Unravelling how the menstrual cycle influences emotions. (2024, March 20). Importikaah. https://importikaah.com/blogs/news/the-hidden-link-unraveling-how-the-menstrual-cycle-influences-emotions

Higginson, C. (2023, May 1).*What is womb healing and why is it so important for creatives?.* Chamonix Higginson. https://www.chahigginson.com/blog/womb-healing-for-creatives

Hoover, A. (2023, July 17). *How to redefine society's view of periods.* Helping Women Period. https://www.helpingwomenperiod.org/redefining_periods/

Hopper, H. (2021, April 6). *Eat, move, and live with your cycle.* Wholistically Hannah https://www.wholisticallyhannah.com/all/how-to-cycle-sync

Hopler, W. (2019, January 3). *Sacred roses: The spiritual symbolism of roses.* Learn Religions. https://www.learnreligions.com/sacred-roses-spiritual-symbolism-rose-123989

How are period tracking apps changing the game for women's health management? (n.d.). Women Tech. https://www.womentech.net/en-at/how-to/how-are-period-tracking-apps-changing-game-womens-health-management

How do you encourage open communication within your family? [Online forum post]. (n.d.). Quora. https://www.quora.com/How-do-you-encourage-open-communication-within-your-family

How to set up a community group successfully. (n.d.). Third Sector Protect. https://www.thirdsectorprotect.co.uk/blog/starting-a-community-group/

Huxter, M. (n.d.). *Insight and Vipassana meditation: Where the attention goes.* Insight Timer. https://insighttimer.com/blog/what-is-insight-meditation/

Importance of menstrual hygiene education for girls in India. (2024, April 13). Cry. https://www.cry.org/blog/importance-of-menstrual-hygiene-education-for-girls-in-india/

Jay, S. (n.d.). *The four female archetypes & how to work with them.* Revoloon. https://revoloon.com/shanijay/the-four-female-archetypes

Jaylyn (2021, July 8). *The #1 menstruation ritual I share with all womben.* Innerswim. https://www.innerswim.com/menstruation-ritual/

Kacane, I., & Hernàndez-Serrano, M. J. (2023). Social connection when physically isolated: Family experiences in using video calls. *Open Cultural Studies, 7*(1). https://doi.org/10.1515/culture-2022-0165

Lindberg, S. (2020, September 23). *The benefits of restorative yoga and poses to try.* Healthline. https://www.healthline.com/health/restorative-yoga-poses

Lorenzana, C. (2023, September 18). *Rituals for each phase of the cycle.* Carmen Lorenzana. https://www.carmenlorenzana.com/2023/05/22/rituals-for-each-phase/

Lynette. (n.d.). *Tree pose benefits and why it is the ideal yoga pose to try.* SweatBox Yoga. https://www.sweatboxyoga.com.sg/tree-pose-yoga/

Maintaining your digital community. (n.d.). eActivities. https://eactivities.union.ic.ac.uk/training/articles/489?collection=90

Mandal, A. (2023, July 7). *What does the uterus do?.* News-Medical.net. https://www.news-medical.net/health/What-Does-the-Uterus-Do.aspx

Martin. N. (n.d.). *Meet your cycle archetypes: The rebel/the maiden.* Natalie K Martin. https://www.nataliekmartin.com/blog/themaidentherebel

McHugh, M. (2020). Menstrual shame: Exploring the role of 'menstrual moaning.' In C. Bobel, I. T. Winkler, B. K. Fahs, A. Hasson, E. A. Kissling, & T.-A. Roberts, *The Palgrave handbook of critical menstruation studies*. Palgrave Macmillan.

Menstrual cycle awareness: The ultimate empowerment tool for women. (n.d.). The Yoga Barn. https://www.theyogabarn.com/blog/menstrual-cycle-awareness.html

Menstrual taboos and ancient wisdom. (2014, March 26). Mythri Speaks. https://mythrispeaks.wordpress.com/2014/03/26/menstrual-taboos-and-ancient-wisdom/

Mindful Staff. (2023, January 6). *Mindfulness meditation: How to do it*. Mindful. https://www.mindful.org/mindfulness-how-to-do-it/

The Minds Journal. (2023, May 22). 7 reasons why mutual understanding is more important than love in a relationship [Image attached] [Post]. LinkedIn. https://www.linkedin.com/pulse/7-reasons-why-mutual-understanding-more-important-than

Naarica. (2023, December 5). *Navigating your partner's menstrual cycle: A guide to support and understanding* [Image attached] [Post]. LinkedIn. https://www.linkedin.com/pulse/navigating-your-partners-menstrual-cycle-guide-support-understanding-dpnef

Nash, J. (2024, February 29). *What is loving-kindness meditation?* Positive Psychology.

https://positivepsychology.com/loving-kindness-meditation/

Natural rhythms: Embracing nature's rhythms: The essence of seasonality. (2024, March 9). Faster Capital. https://fastercapital.com/content/Natural-rhythms—Embracing-Nature-s-Rhythms—The-Essence-of-Seasonality.html

Niculet, D. (2022, March 8). *Essential oils for the 4 phases of the menstrual cycle.* The Oil Stories. https://www.theoilstories.com/blogs/news/essential-oils-for-each-of-the-4-stages-of-the-menstrual-cycle

Nunez, K. (n.d.). *How to: Talk to your partner about mental health & your period.* Marea. https://mareawellness.com/blogs/news/how-to-talk-to-your-partner-about-mental-health-your-period

Onega, S (2021). *The symbolization of the female body in western culture from ancient Greece to the transmodern period.* In R. Ahrens, F. Klaeger, & K. Stierstorfer (Eds.), *Symbolism: An international annual of critical aesthetics.* De Gruyter.

Pacheco, D., & Callender, E. (2024, March 12). *Women & sleep: Needs, disorders, & recommendations.* Sleep Foundation. https://www.sleepfoundation.org/women-sleep

Parsley Health. (2023, May 26). *What to eat during your menstrual cycle phases.* Cora. https://cora.life/blogs/blood-milk/what-to-eat-during-your-menstrual-cycle-phases

The power of the PEP rally. (n.d.). Period Education Project. https://periodeducationproject.org/community-events/

Providence Health Team. (n.d.). *One woman's story: Staying grounded, resilient in adversity.* Providence. https://blog.providence.org/blog/one-woman-s-story-staying-grounded-resilient-in-adversity

Rabins, A. (n.d.). *Suggestions for a first menstruation celebration.* Ritualwell. https://ritualwell.org/ritual/suggestions-first-menstruation-celebration/

Relationships and communication. (n.d.). Better Health Channel. https://www.betterhealth.vic.gov.au/health/healthyliving/relationships-and-communication

Resende, L (2023, August 3). *Sisterhood. Real women, real stories. Marisol Kiyoko and resilience* [Image attached] [Post]. LinkedIn. https://www.linkedin.com/pulse/sisterhood-real-women-stories-marisol-kiyoko-let%C3%ADcia-resende

The ritual & benefits of yoni steaming. (2023, February 9). Make & Mary https://makeandmary.com/blogs/blog/the-ritual-benefits-of-yoni-steaming

Rituals to start cycle syncing: Aligning your lifestyle with your menstrual phases. (n.d.). Xula Herbs. https://www.xulaherbs.com/blogs/blog/rituals-to-start-cycle-syncing-aligning-your-lifestyle-with-your-menstrual-phases

Rizopoulos, N., & Long, R. (2024, March 23). *Mountain pose.* Yoga Journal. https://www.yogajournal.com/poses/mountain-pose/

Ryan, A. (2023, May 07). *Reclaiming spirit.* https://ugc.production.linktr.ee/843d00f1-af64-48ca-839c-13e806176e9f_Reclaiming-Spirit-Workbook.pdf

Samira. (2024, February 19). *Period pride: Why loving your period matters.* SageSistas. https://sagesistas.com/period-health-why-loving-your-period-matters/

Social Tables. (n.d.). *15 community event ideas that bring people together.* Cvent. https://www.socialtables.com/blog/event-planning/community-event-ideas/

Stark, M. (2021, June 23). *Our rhythm is our cycle.* tbd. https://www.tbd.community/en/a/our-rhythm-our-cycle

Stirling, K . (n.d.). *Inner seasons.* Kellie Stirling. https://www.kelliestirling.com/innerseasons

Suff, R. & McCartney, C. (2023, December 8). *Building momentum for menstrual health support.* Chartered Institute of Personnel and Development. https://www.cipd.org/en/views-and-insights/thought-leadership/cipd-voice/menstrual-health-support/

Supporting menstrual health and hygiene to improve women and girls' wellbeing. (n.d.). Engender Health. https://www.engenderhealth.org/article/supporting-menstrual-health-and-hygiene-to-improve-women-and-girls-wellbeing

Support system: how family and friends shape our lives. (2024, April 19). Faster Capital. https://fastercapital.com/content/Support-System—How-Family-and-Friends-Shape-our-Lives.html

Tajiri, N. (2019, May 3). *She dreams when she bleeds: Poems about periods.* Independently published.

Team Hummingway. (2021, October 19). *Talking to your partner about your cycle.* Hummingway. https://ourhummingway.com/article/talking-to-your-partner-about-your-cycle

10 ways to show your partner appreciation. (n.d.). Centerstone. https://centerstone.org/our-resources/health-wellness/10-ways-to-show-your-partner-appreciation/

Unlocking community insights: Strategies for effective engagement. (2024, April 2). Faster Capital. https://fastercapital.com/content/Community-insights-Unlocking-Community-Insights—Strategies-for-Effective-Engagement.html

Waldorf, S, & Grollemond, L. (2024, March 4). *Getting your period in the Middle Ages.* Getty. https://www.getty.edu/news/education-periods-facts-women-medieval-history-past-before-pads-tampons/

Walter, M. (2021, September 1). *Is there really a connection between your menstrual cycle and the moon?* Healthline. https://www.healthline.com/health/womens-health/menstrual-cycle-and-the-moon

Ward, F. (2022, April 12). *'Mindful menstruation' is the latest wellness trend combining your period and mindfulness – here's how it works.* Glamour. https://www.glamourmagazine.co.uk/article/how-mindful-menstruation-can-change-your-periods

WebMD Editorial Contributors. (n.d.-a). *What are biological rhythms?* WebMD. https://www.webmd.com/a-to-z-guides/what-are-biological-rhythms

WebMD Editorial Contributors. (n.d.-b). *What is breathwork?* https://www.webmd.com/balance/what-is-breathwork

What is menstruation awareness? (n.d.). Raleigh OB/GYN. https://www.raleighob.com/what-is-menstruation-awareness/

Whitman, L. (n.d.). *Why staying connected with family is essential for seniors and how to do it.* Memory Cherish. https://memorycherish.com/staying-connected-with-family/

Willemaine-Green, C.(2020, June 24). *22 sacred rituals for honoring your menstrual cycle.* Earth Daughters. https://www.earthdaughters.org/library/womb-menstruation-blood-rituals

Wisner, W. (2024a, January 29). *Everything you need to know about the luteal phase of your menstrual cycle.* Health. https://www.health.com/luteal-phase-8425312

Wisner, W. (2024b, March 15). *Should I try cycle syncing? Here's what the experts say.* Verywell Mind.

https://www.verywellmind.com/cycle-syncing-for-well-being-8597591

Wright, G., & Yasar, K. (n.d.). *What is social networking?* Tech Target https://www.techtarget.com/whatis/definition/social-networking

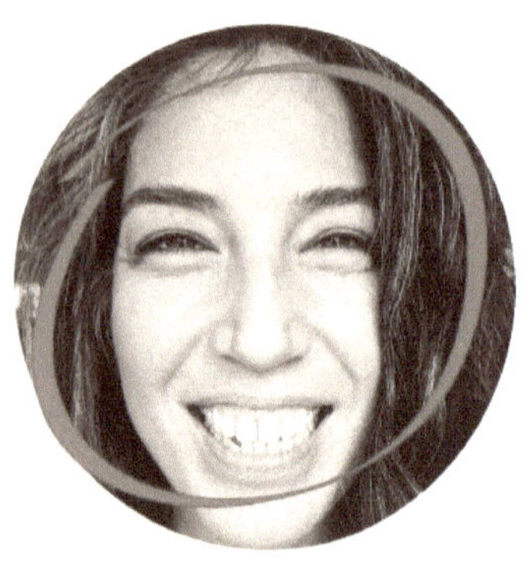

About the Author

Eda Gungor (Pen name I AM EDA) is a renowned wellness advocate and mentor, celebrated for her holistic approach to empowering women. With over a decade of experience in the wellness industry, Eda has developed numerous transformative programs, retreats, and workshops, and authored this insightful book along with others. As the visionary founder of SEVA Experience, she leads a pioneering wellness hub that includes an acclaimed plant-based café and a conscious living store. Eda's work is dedicated to helping individuals claim their power and embrace their unapologetic selves. Through her offerings, she serves as the spark that ignites profound growth and empowerment.

Read more at https://www.iameda.com/.